HOMOEOPATH

Revised Edition

Homoeopathic Prescribing

Revised Edition

Dr Noel J. Pratt
MRCS, LRCP, FFHom

With an Appendix on the Constitutional Remedies
by Dr Marion Gray, BM, BCh, MRCGP, MFHom

BEACONSFIELD PUBLISHERS LTD
Beaconsfield, Bucks, England

First published in 1980
Reprinted 1981
Revised Edition 1985
Reprinted 1991

British Library Cataloguing in Publication Data

Pratt, Noel J.
   Homoeopathic prescribing. – (Beaconsfield
   homoeopathic library; No. 3).
   1. Homeopathy – Materia medica and therapeutics
   2. Drugs – Prescribing
   I. Title
   615.532   RX601

ISBN 0–906584–03–5

Phototypeset in 9½ on 10 point Times.
Printed in Great Britain at The Bath Press, Avon.

Dedicated to the memory of
Francis Hervey Bodman,
MD, ChB, MRCS, LRCP, FRCPsych, DPM, FFHom
in gratitude for his many writings.

INTRODUCTION

This book is intended for the student of homoeopathy who requires short lists of remedies for most of the common ailments.

In composing these lists I have referred to the works of other authors, in addition to drawing on my own experience of homoeopathic prescribing in thirty years in the National Health Service. I gratefully acknowledge my main sources of reference:

Dr C. M. Boger's *Synoptic Key of the Materia Medica*, Dr J. H. Clarke's *The Prescriber*, Dr D. M. Gibson's *Homoeopathic First Aid*, Dr R. Hughes' *Principles and Practice of Homoeopathy*, Dr J. T. Kent's *Repertory*, Drs Neatby and Stonham's *Manual of Homoeopathic Therapeutics* and Dr Margaret Tyler's *Drug Pictures*.

This book is primarily for qualified physicians, who will know when investigation and other treatment is needed. The book can, of course, be bought by others who are not medically qualified but require the information for the benefit of themselves, their families and friends. To such persons I say: homoeopathy is of great value as first aid and for minor diseases, but if there is any doubt of the significance of the symptoms and signs of the disease for which a remedy is sought, be sure to obtain the opinion of a qualified physician. You may find the homoeopathic remedy a valuable supplement to other treatment.

The list of symptoms, signs and diagnoses is presented in alphabetical order. The sections are confined to one page for ease of reference and to avoid any confusion which might arise from long lists of remedies, including some which are seldom used. In each section the remedies are presented in alphabetical order; this is better than trying to arrange them in order of importance, about which opinions would differ. Lay terms are not always included – sometimes they are deliberately omitted. For example, 'Spots' would be an unsatisfactory section; the prescriber must know what variety of spots is in question. Relatively vague terms such as Sore Throat have no separate sections, because the reader will need to make a more precise diagnosis, such as

Tonsillitis, Pharyngitis, Laryngitis, or Tracheitis, and then refer to the appropriate page.

I have carefully considered the suggestion that the subject matter should be presented under the headings of the anatomical systems most involved in each disease. I have decided not to do so, because the book does not pretend to be a systematic textbook in that sense, but essentially a handbook for quick refreshing of the memory.

The brief notes after each remedy will not always be sufficient to select the right one without further thought; these few symptoms and signs are in the nature of reminders, to encourage further thought. It is usually necessary to take into account not only the main symptoms and signs, but also the physical and temperamental characteristics of the patient, and the various factors which make the disease better or worse.

Critics may object that the presentation of short lists of remedies will encourage prescribers to dodge the work of formal repertorisation on paper in the Kentian manner. There are times when full repertorisation is necessary, but there are other times when personal experience enables a simpler way of selecting the similimum, especially when aided by a handbook such as this.

It will be noticed that there are only a few sections concerning mental symptoms and the various moods and temperaments. The main reason is that to include them all would make the book unwieldy. In Kent's *Repertory*, for example, there are eighty-four major rubrics in the ninety-four pages devoted to 'Mind'. Therefore no attempt has been made to mention all of them.

Strange, rare and peculiar symptoms are mentioned, just as in the clinical situation patients sometimes describe their troubles in strange, rare and peculiar terms. In teaching hospitals these are usually ignored because they do not fit into the textbook descriptions of disease. Many doctors hardly hear them because they seem to be irrelevant to prescribing, but when they are used for selecting the homoeopathic remedy, their value is great.

The list of subjects is deliberately not comprehensive; most of the infectious, contagious and notifiable diseases have been omitted, because if they are not treated (and when necessary notified) on conventional lines, allegations of negligence are possible. Nevertheless, homoeopathic remedies can be valuable additional treatment, especially in convalescence and for any sequelae.

Homoeopathy cannot, in my opinion, reverse degenerative diseases, but experience of its use does seem to justify the hope that it may restrain degenerative processes or even halt them, by improving the general health.

Dr Marion Gray's list of constitutional remedies and the main indications for them is a welcome Appendix to the book. Whenever no 'local' or 'organ' remedy is clearly indicated, reference to the list of constitutional remedies will usually enable the choice to be made with confidence.

I am grateful to my friends Dr Hamish Boyd, Dr David Gemmell, Dr Marianne Harling, Dr Alastair Jack, Dr Marion Gray and Mr John Ainsworth, MPS, all of whom read and made many helpful comments on earlier or later drafts for the book.

Homoeopathic knowledge continues to grow, as is shown by the recent publication of the *Materia Medica of New Homoeopathic Remedies* by Dr O. A. Julian of Paris, in which there are seventy-eight new remedies described and recent additional information about twenty-eight other remedies.

Every homoeopath should strive to record all that he or she learns from experience, as well as from conversations and from reading. The interleaved pages of this book are suitable for recording such knowledge.

N.J.P.

POTENCY AND DOSAGE

In response to several requests, I venture to offer advice on the subject of potency and dosage. It is not easy to do this – there are no fixed rules, and each prescriber works in ways based on his or her teaching, study, and experience.

There are many factors which influence the decision on which potency and what dosage to use; the nature of the disease, the patient's physique and temperament and reactions to various circumstances, the previous treatment, necessary concurrent treatment, and the patient's knowledge of homoeopathic medicine. In tailoring terms, 'made to measure' is needed for the best results.

It is nevertheless possible to offer the reader a number of generally agreed principles for the administration of homoeopathic remedies, and the following guidelines are an attempt to summarise the practice of the majority of homoeopathic physicians.

Potency

Low potencies are those in which some of the original substance of the remedy is still present. They are generally available as 3x, 6x, 6c and 12c. They have wide application, are less likely to cause aggravations, and the beginner is advised to use them, especially as they are the potencies most likely to be available at local pharmacies.

High potencies are those in which there are no molecules of the remedy remaining – only the homoeopathic potency, which is still a mystery from the biophysical point of view, but clinically effective, often producing remarkable results. The high potencies are best prescribed by the more experienced physicians.

As a general rule, the low potencies are indicated for diseases which are localised, and not affecting the patient's general health. The high potencies are usually indicated when the patient's general health is disturbed, and also when the disease has a predominantly psychological cause.

Constitutional remedies (such as those listed in Dr Gray's Appendix) are usually prescribed in the 30c and the higher potencies. Nosodes (equivalent to oral vaccines in potency) should also be prescribed in high potency, 200c or higher.

When a low potency brings some improvement which is followed by a relapse, a higher potency of the same remedy is often indicated, and can be expected to work deeper and longer.

Dosage

The ideal cure is achieved by one dose of a single remedy; this does happen, if the dose is given time to work. When first-aid is needed for injuries, a single dose is usually enough. The long-term sequelae of trauma in the broadest sense of the word are also often eliminated by a single dose, but the physician must be prepared to repeat the remedy to maintain the improvement or cure.

Sometimes the single dose is given 'split' – half in the evening and half the next morning, on the assumption that the body may respond to the stimulus better at one time of the day than at another. In other cases a succession of doses may be needed to stimulate the system to respond, especially when the patient is elderly. Some patients are unduly sensitive to medicaments, and then it is wise to begin treatment with one dose on the first day, two on the second day, and then three times a day – using low potencies – until improvement is noticed, and then to stop and review the situation.

Acute diseases. In very acute circumstances, such as the onset of a fever, doses may be given at short but increasing intervals such as one, two, four and eight hours. After that, a second remedy may be needed for the second stage of the illness. This applies particularly to the common infectious diseases of childhood, when the symptoms and signs change.

Subacute diseases. Some, such as lingering respiratory catarrh or sinusitis, often need a course of a remedy twice a day for a few days, and occasionally longer.

Chronic diseases usually need higher potencies which work deeper and longer. Then a dose of a high potency such as the 30c can be given once a week until improvement is established. Some prescribers begin treatment of chronic disease with a single dose of the constitutional remedy in high potency, followed by a course of a low potency of the 'organ' remedy for the organ or system most affected. Or, the organ remedy in low potency (3x, 6x or 6c) may be used daily or twice daily six days each week, and the constitutional remedy in high potency on the seventh day of each week.

Episodic diseases, such as migraine, can be treated with one dose at the onset of the attack. If this is found to cause an aggravation, the remedy should be withheld till after an attack. Some chronic diseases are exacerbated in a fairly regular and predictable time of day or week or month, or at certain times of the menstrual cycle; then it is advisable to give a dose on the day before an expected attack. For premenstrual tension, the remedy can be given when symptoms appear, expecting to need fewer doses each month, and eventually none at all.

Before and after surgical operations it is usually appropriate to give a dose before going into hospital, and another on return home.

Prophylaxis. For the prevention of influenza, and for building up immunity to other infections such as some of the childhood fevers, three doses of the nosode at intervals of one week are usually enough. Some physicians prescribe a dose at monthly intervals throughout the winter in those who are particularly susceptible. Nosodes should not be given during an attack of the infection concerned. When convalescence is slow, one or two doses of the appropriate nosode or the constitutional remedy are indicated.

Administration of the Remedy. Unless the symptoms are very urgent, it is preferable to give the remedy between meals, not less than thirty minutes before or after food. Any unnatural taste in the mouth, such as tobacco, alcoholic drink, coffee, or toothpaste, lozenges, or commercial 'sweets', should be washed away by a thorough rinsing of the mouth with plain water or with one of the natural spring waters.

Homoeopathic remedies are best absorbed through the mucosal lining of the mouth – so the tablets, pills, granules, or powders should be retained in the mouth until they have dissolved. Some tablets which dissolve slowly may be chewed after half to one minute.

CONTENTS

ACNE

In addition to the usual advice on diet, skin care and general hygiene, these remedies should be considered:

Belladonna   for acne in full-blooded, red-faced persons.

Hepar Sul.   when pustules are a prominent feature.

Pulsatilla   for acne in pale blondes of either sex.

Silica   when there is much scarring.

Staphylococcin   if the response to other remedies is slow.

Sulphur   for long-standing obstinate cases.

ACNE ROSACEA

Arsenicum Album   when there is noticeable desquamation and burning sensations.

Belladonna   for full-blooded, red-faced persons.

Lachesis   when caused by oral contraceptives; in addition to the eruption, there is burning of the face, worse in hot rooms and worse after taking alcohol.

Nux Vomica   when there is an above-average intake of alcohol, especially of spirits.

Rhus Tox.   when the nose is red, shiny and swollen, and there is a tendency to develop pustules.

Sulphur Iod.   when the face is dry and red, and develops pustules.

ADENOIDS, ENLARGED

Bacillinum   when there is a family tendency to enlarged adenoids, and especially if there is a family history of tuberculosis.

Barium Carb.   for children who are under-developed physically and also mentally backward.

Calc. Carb.   for pale, fat children with cold, clammy feet, and sweating of the head at night.

Calc. Phos.   for thin children with large troublesome adenoids.

Psorinum   with itchy skin and offensive sweat.

Sulphur   for the child who is always hungry, especially about eleven in the morning, and has a marked dislike of hot baths; for adenoids (and tonsils) which are so large as to cause some degree of obstruction.

AGGRESSION

Belladonna   for sudden and violent aggression, with an 'inclination' to bite.

Nux Vomica   when the patient is easily offended, reacts irritably, and develops tension headaches and dyspepsia.

Sepia   for the occasional episodes of aggression in contrast to the usual depression and apathy.

Staphisagria   when aggressive tendencies arise from resentment or anger which is more or less repressed, with consequent physical repercussions.

Sulphur   for persons with aggressive tendencies concerning institutions rather than people – social reformers with strange, even grandiose, ideas: 'burning with zeal, and itching for action'.

ALCOHOLISM

Some form of psychotherapy is always needed, as well as advice on diet and habits.

Aconite   for episodes of fear and delirium.

Antim. Tart.   for nausea and vomiting, especially if there is also bronchial catarrh.

Arsenicum Album   for restlessness and mental aberrations.

Capsicum   when the main symptom is gastritis.

Cinchona   wants to be alone for solitary drinking.

Crotalus Horridus   when vomiting of blood occurs. (That may necessitate admission to hospital.)

Lachesis   for the voluble social over-drinker.

Nux Vomica   for hangovers and morning vomiting, especially after brandy.

Quercus   to help to suppress the craving.

Sulphur   will drink almost anything, indiscriminately.

Tuberculinum   when drinking leads to violence.

Zinc Met.   with twitching and trembling.

ANGER, AND AILMENTS AFTER ANGER

Aconite   for anger originating in fright – for example, the situation after a road accident.

Chamomilla   for anger in the young, and in the old – the remedy for cantankerous behaviour in 'second childhood'.

Colocynth   for anger leading to colic and neuralgia.

Crocus   for anger with violence, with quick repentance.

Hepar Sul.   easily roused to vehemence and rapid speech.

Ignatia   unreasonable anger leading to a variety of hysterical manifestations.

Nux Vomica   irritability and anger, causing dyspepsia and other troubles.

Staphisagria   suppressed anger and indignation, leading to headaches and other pains.

ANGINA PECTORIS

Aconite   when the pain causes much alarm, and especially if there is also tingling in the arm or hand.

Cactus   with the classical sensation of an iron band round the chest, 'as in a vice'.

Carbo Veg.   for pseudo-angina, caused by excess wind in the stomach, or by too big a meal.

Glonoine   with much throbbing.

Lachesis   with a sense of constriction in the neck as well as in the chest.

Latrodectus   with rapid pulse, nausea and vomiting.

Lilium Tig.   when the heart feels squeezed, alternately grasped and relaxed.

Spigelia   with marked palpitations, noticeable to observers.

ANUS, FISSURE OF

Aesculus   with burning soreness and pain in the back.

Chamomilla   with haemorrhoids.

Graphites   with painful smarting and soreness.

Nitric Acid   with sharp cutting pains and prickings.

Ratanhia   with burning after defaecation, and sharp stabs as if with a knife.

Silica   when healing is slow.

Thuja   with various other anal and rectal symptoms and pain causing frequency of micturition.

Tuberculinum   with a sense of pressure in the rectum and leading to diarrhoea.

ANUS, ITCHING OF (PRURITIS ANI)

Alumina   with prickling as if by pins.

Ambra Grisea   with itching of the pudenda.

Antim. Crud.   with smarting, worse at night.

Ignatia   with violent itching and crawling sensations, but not due to threadworms.

Nitric Acid   worse when walking in the open air, and after stool.

Petroleum   worse when riding in cars, and worse at night in bed.

Sulphur   with prolapse of the anus as well as the itching.

3

APPETITE, CRAVINGS

Argentum Nit. for sweet things and salty things.

Calc. Carb. for salt.

Carbo Anim. for sour and refreshing items of diet.

China for something, but does not know what.

Hepar Sul. for sour or highly flavoured pungent things such as curry.

Ignatia for indigestible things, especially in pregnancy.

Natrum Mur. for salt.

Nux Vomica for brandy.

Phosphorus for sugar, but not for fats.

Psorinum appetite much increased for anything.

Pulsatilla for beer.

Sepia for vinegar.

Silica for cold uncooked foods.

Sulphur for fats and for sugar.

APPETITE, LOSS OF

Calc. Carb. especially does not want meat.

Ignatia loss of appetite for everything.

Nux Vomica appetite spoilt by bitter taste in the mouth, and a tongue with a thick yellow coating.

Lycopodium fullness after a few mouthfuls, as if too much has already been eaten.

Pulsatilla little appetite, and no thirst.

Rhus Tox. loss of appetite for everything.

APPREHENSION

Argentum Nit. apprehension leading to diarrhoea.

Arsenicum Album with restlessness – paces up and down.

Carbo Veg. especially on waking – and wants fresh air.

Gelsemium unable to act – 'paralysed' by apprehension.

Lycopodium dreads tasks like making speeches, but when the time comes, rises to the occasion.

Medorrhinum with the feeling that time goes too slowly.

Phosphoric Acid a mixture of apprehension and indifference.

Plumbum with impaired memory, and fear of forgetting words.

Silica with undue sensitivity to music.

Thuja with headache like a nail being driven into the head.

4

ARTHRITIS, ACUTE

Apis with much swelling of the soft tissues, and redness, like a bee sting.

Arnica especially helpful when arthritic joints are bruised by blows and falls.

Bryonia for acute exacerbations, when no relief is obtained from movement – in contrast to Rhus Tox.

Dulcamara when noticeably worse after cold and damp, as from unaired beds, as well as from damp weather.

Ledum after injections – when corticosteroid injections have not been as helpful as expected.

Pulsatilla pains go from joint to joint, and are variable and unpredictable.

ARTHRITIS, CHRONIC

Argentum Nit. for the anxious person who tends to move too fast and has accidents which aggravate the arthritis.

Aurum Met. in homoeopathic potency, as valuable as the conventional injections, and without risk of dermatitis.

Calc. Fluor. when exostoses develop in association with arthritis.

Calc. Phos. when arthritis is initiated or made worse during pregnancy.

Causticum especially when contractures develop or threaten.

Colchicum for gouty arthritis.

Kali Bich. for joint pains alternating with catarrhal or gastric symptoms.

Nux Vomica for associated muscle spasms as distinct from muscle stiffness.

Rhus Tox. when there is muscle stiffness protecting the affected joints – better after moving about a little.

Ruta when ganglia are present.

Sepia for menopausal arthritis.

Sulphur for psoriatic arthritis.

ASTHMA

It is impossible to condense the many remedies for asthma on to one page, but a short list may be helpful. In addition to the constitutional remedies and the nosodes the following should be considered:

Antim. Tart. with wheezing so loud that it can be heard in the next room.

Arsenicum Album with restlessness.

Ipecacuanha with catarrh of the nose and throat, and with scanty sputum.

Kali Carb. especially if attacks begin between 3 a.m. and 5 a.m.

Lobelia with nausea and a tendency to heart failure.

Natrum Sul. when there is a tendency to salt and water retention and morning diarrhoea, and the asthma is worse in damp weather.

Veratrum Viride when a condition similar to shock develops – cold sweat, nausea and vomiting.

BACKACHE

These are a few of the many remedies which are valuable for back pain and also for associated weakness of the back.

Arnica for bruises and for sensations similar to bruises.

Arsenicum Album backache with restlessness – cannot find a comfortable position.

Calc. Carb. worse while sitting.

Kali Carb. for backache and weakness persisting after pregnancy and labour.

Nux Vomica with tension in the back muscles, limiting flexion of the spine.

Phosphoric Acid when weakness is more complained of than pain.

Rhus Tox. if stiffness is marked, especially on first movements, and better after continued movement.

BELCHING

Argentum Nit.   loud copious and painless belching.

Carbo An.   with a sense of pressure, and with choking.

Carbo Veg.   with distension of the stomach.

Carbolic Acid   with nervous dyspepsia.

Mag. Carb.   with vomiting of sour fluid.

Mag. Phos.   small belches without relief of discomfort.

Mancinella   with burning sensations rising from the stomach to the throat.

Phosphorus   desires cold drinks.

Pulsatilla   belching with a taste of the food of the last meal.

Sulphur   belching with particles of food and with an unpleasant smell.

BLEPHARITIS

Apis   for acute cases with much redness, burning, stinging, and swelling of the eyelids.

Belladonna   also for the acute stage, especially if the eyes are dry and hot, and the pupils are dilated.

Hepar Sul.   when the eyelids are stuck together after sleep, and when the pain threshold is low.

Merc. Sol.   when there is much exudate, and when blepharo-spasm is pronounced.

BLISTERS AND VESICLES

Arsenicum Album   burning sensations, better for warmth.

Cantharis   for burns and scalds to prevent the development of blisters.

Causticum   for vesicles, fissures and warts – with a raw feeling, as if the skin were grazed.

Lachesis   vesicles with a purple or blue tinge, leaving ulcers, especially on the left.

Mezereum   especially when the scalp is involved and when thick scabs are formed.

Natrum Mur.   for blisters or vesicles on the lips.

Nitric Acid   with pricking sensations.

Phosphorus   with burning sensations and fidgeting.

Ranunculus   for shingles on the chest wall.

Rhus Tox.   when urticaria is severe and the lesions almost look like blisters.

BOILS AND FURUNCLES

Diabetes and other causes should be detected or excluded in case other treatment is essential. Then the following remedies may be considered:

Apis   with much redness and swelling around the boil.

Arnica   for boils in sensitive parts, with bruised sensation.

Arsenicum Album   with burning sensations.

Belladonna   when boils are surrounded by bright red 'angry' areas.

Graphites   with dry skin, and insufficient sweat to keep it healthy.

Hepar Sul.   when every little skin injury turns septic and when blisters develop into boils.

Lachesis   unusually painful boils with a bluish tinge.

Merc. Sol.   for furuncles in the ears.

Phytolacca   for boils on the back.

Pyrogen   for angry spreading boils.

Silica   for boils which develop slowly and heal slowly, especially in chilly persons.

Staphylococcin   for furunculosis.

Sulphur   when a series of boils occurs, especially if the patient scratches a lot.

Tarentula   purplish boils with severe burning and stinging.

BONE PAINS

Aurum Met.   burning and boring pains in bones, with redness and swelling – if it has been proved *not* to be due to osteomyelitis.

Eupatorium   bone pains during influenza.

Hekla Lava   painful lumps on bones – exostoses.

Kali Bich.   for pains in small spots, especially in or on the bones of the head.

Mezereum   rheumatic pains in bones, worse at night.

Phosphorus   burning pains in bones, especially of the mandible – similar to the 'phossy jaw' of phosphorus poisoning.

Rhododendron   worse before stormy weather – for persons who can thus foretell rain and thunder.

Ruta   pains associated with sprains.

Silica   for children who are thin and weak and complain of bone pains.

BREAST, PAIN IN

Asterias Rubens   for drawing pains associated with cancer – as supplementary treatment.

Belladonna   with throbbing.

Bellis Perennis   also for pain of breast cancer.

Bryonia   with heaviness, better for gentle pressure and support.

Calc. Carb.   pain before periods.

Conium   pain before periods, with lumpiness.

Graphites   for painful cracked nipples, in addition to local treatment.

Hepar Sul.   when slight injuries lead to suppuration or inflammation.

Lachesis   pains worse on waking.

Merc. Sol.   pains worse at night.

Phytolacca   for mastitis, with the characteristic swelling and lumpiness.

Pulsatilla   for pains which come and go unpredictably, causing tears.

Silica   undue pain while nursing the baby.

BRONCHITIS

Aconite   in the early stages.

Ammon. Carb.   in the later stages, when it is difficult to raise the sputum.

Antim. Tart.   when there is loud rattling in the chest.

Arsenicum Album   worse at night – with much coughing but little sputum.

Belladonna   in the early stages, with hot dry skin and red face.

Bryonia   dry hacking cough with pain in the chest.

Carbo Veg.   for older persons with a tendency to cyanosis.

Causticum   with stress incontinence of urine.

Conium   short dry cough with tickling behind the sternum.

Hepar Sul.   with profuse yellow sputum.

Hyoscyamus   the cough begins as soon as the patient lies down.

Ipecacuanha   cough leading to nausea and gagging.

Kali Bich.   when the sputum is tenacious and stringy.

Merc. Sol.   with a tendency to extra sweating.

Pulsatilla   worse lying down and in a warm room.

Rumex   with soreness in the trachea and behind the sternum; worse in cold air.

Senega   for painful rattling in the chest – sputum hard to raise.

Stannum   bronchitis with a weak feeling in the chest.

Sulphur   for the later stages of bronchitis, when the cough is worse in bed at night.

BRUISES

Arnica   the remedy most often used for bruises, especially when muscles are involved.

Bellis   for bruises of the breast.

Hamamelis   when the skin over a bruise is broken, also for bruises of varicose veins.

Hypericum   for bruises of parts especially rich in nerve endings – the fingers and toes.

Ruta   for injuries involving bruises of bones and of tendons.

BUNIONS

Antim. Crud.   for elderly persons with tender feet, worse in warm rooms.

Benzoic Acid   especially for persons with gout as well as bunions.

Kali Iod.   when there is also a tendency to chilblains.

Rhododendron   when bunions are more painful before storms.

Silica   when the bunions are hard and not much inflamed.

BURNS AND SCALDS

Cantharis   usually the best first aid, in the form of lotion.

Causticum   for painful burn scars.

Hamamelis   can also be used as a lotion as first aid.

Hepar Sul.   for burns which have become infected.

Kali Bich.   for second degree burns – the equivalent of ulcers.

Urtica   for persistent stinging sensations.

CATARRH, CHRONIC NASAL

Obstinate cases often require constitutional remedies as **Pulsatilla, Sulphur, Psorinum, Tuberculinum, Carcinosinum** and **Morgan Co**. These remedies are usually chosen on the personal history, but at other times the family history is of value in deciding which is needed.

Arsenicum Iod. in weakly debilitated persons with drippy nose and sore nostrils.

Aurum Met. with soreness of the nasal bones, and much depression.

Graphites when there is also constipation, and skin eruptions around the nostrils.

Hydrastis for constant post-nasal drip and eustachian catarrh.

Kali Bich. with yellow or white stringy catarrh.

Natrum Mur. fluent catarrh, intermittent, variable in quantity from day to day; much sneezing.

Sanguinaria with stinging and tickling in the nose, and some swelling, inside and outside.

CHICKEN POX

In addition to the usual nursing care, the following remedies should be considered:

Antim. Crud. the patient cries if washed or touched, or even if looked at.

Antim. Tart. wants much attention and is very irritable.

Pulsatilla weeps easily; has little thirst.

Rhus Tox. with itching and restlessness; to encourage the drying of the vesicles.

Sulphur hot, eats little but drinks lots.

One can also consider treatment in a sequential scheme:

Aconite in the initial stages.

Rhus Tox. when the blisters form.

Merc. Sol. during convalescence.

Varicellinum when sequelae persist.

CHILBLAINS

Agaricus   more painful when cold.

Apis   with stinging sensations, even when they are not in contact with anything.

Arsenicum Album   with burning sensations.

Calc. Carb.   in pale and obese persons, better when cold.

Graphites   for broken chilblains, with a gluey exudate.

Kali Iod.   when there is much swelling around the chilblains.

Nux Vomica   for persons in sedentary occupations, underweight, and dislike of windy weather.

Petroleum   when the skin has broken – and when the finger tips are cracked.

Pulsatilla   more painful in warm rooms and in bed, and particularly after exposure to radiant heat.

Rhus Tox.   when there is blistering associated with chilblains.

Tamus   when the desire to scratch is irresistible.

Zincum Met.   for chilblains which are worse after rubbing, especially in persons with fidgety feet.

COCCYDYNIA (PAIN IN COCCYX)

Antim. Tart.   with a sensation of a heavy load on the coccyx, dragging the body down.

Apis   burning and stinging pain.

Causticum   drawing or bruised sensation.

Cicuta   tearing and jerking pain.

Hypericum   after a fall.

Kali Bich.   pain worse when sitting and when touched.

Silica   with constipation.

Zincum Met.   with fidgety feet.

COLIC, INTESTINAL

Belladonna with distension of the transverse colon, with relief when 'doubled up'.

Bryonia better when lying still, and worse from heat.

Chamomilla worse at night, especially during teething.

Cina flatulent colic in older children, with or without infestation by worms.

Cocculus flatulent colic during menstruation.

Colocynth sharp 'cutting' colic, better for bending double, can't keep still – writhes and twists.

Dioscerea colic worse for pressure, better for straightening the spine and for walking about.

Mag. Phos. with sharp cramping pains, better for heat.

Plumbum with obstinate constipation and other symptoms similar to lead poisoning.

Stannum when the pain comes on slowly and passes slowly.

Staphisagria colic due to suppressed anger or indignation.

Veratrum Album severe colic leading to symptoms of shock.

COLITIS

These remedies are worth considering for colitis, whether it be mucous colitis, ulcerative colitis or irritable colon.

Argentum Nit. worse when anticipating any kind of ordeal.

Arsenicum Album worse after midnight.

Cantharis with urinary symptoms as well.

Colchicum watery stools.

Colocynth with much colic.

Graphites for obese patients, with offensive flatus.

Kali Sul. worse in the evenings.

Merc. Corr. with blood as well as mucus.

Merc. Sol. with much mucus.

Natrum Sul. worse in the mornings.

Sulphur worse early in the mornings – about 5 a.m.

Veratrum Album copious stools causing faintness.

COMMON COLD

Aconite   in the early stage – in the first night.

Allium Cepa   with much sneezing and watering of the eyes.

Arsenicum Album   with watery catarrh causing sore nostrils.

Euphrasia   with irritating tears but bland nasal catarrh.

Ferrum Phos.   with nose bleeding.

Gelsemium   when the onset is rapid, with chills running up and down the spine.

Hepar Sul.   in later stages when the catarrh is thick and yellow.

Kali Iod.   if the patient is hot and cold alternately, with a red nose and pain in the forehead.

Mag. Mur.   with marked loss of taste and smell.

Mercurius   with much sweating, salivation and thick catarrh.

Natrum Mur.   when there is much sneezing in the morning.

Nux Vomica   fluent nasal catarrh in the day and little at night, and much irritability and intolerance.

Pulsatilla   intermittent catarrh, no thirst and better out of doors.

Sanguinaria   watery catarrh and a tickling dry cough.

Silica   slow onset, slow recovery and with sinusitis.

COMPLEXION

Sometimes a patient's facial appearance is a valuable clue to the choice of a remedy – provided that the symptoms and signs confirm that choice.

Alumina   an unhealthy 'earthy' appearance.

Apis   when the face is swollen and red.

Arsenicum Album   bluish rings around the eyes.

Belladonna   bright red.

Calc. Carb.   pale and wrinkled.

Gelsemium   flushed and congested, with heavy upper eyelids.

Lachesis   distended veins and a cyanotic tinge.

Lycopodium   wrinkled forehead and pale face.

Phosphorus   a 'fresh' red complexion.

Platinum   sallow or 'earthy'.

Sepia   sallow, brown and with darkened eyelids.

Sulphur   red-faced.

Thuja   warts and other lumpy lesions.

Veratrum Album   the 'Hippocratic' facial appearance of shock and collapse.

CONCUSSION

Homoeopathic remedies are valuable as first aid after concussion, and are also valuable for the sequelae.

Arnica   especially when there is visible bruising.

Cicuta   when there are any convulsions or muscle twitchings.

Helleborus   when headache persists and is 'stupefying'.

Hypericum   if the head is extremely sensitive.

Kali Phos.   with insomnia persisting.

Natrum Mur.   when depression persists.

CONJUNCTIVITIS

If there is any doubt concerning the cause of conjunctivitis, the opinion of an ophthalmologist should be obtained. In simple cases, in addition to local treatment, homoeopathic remedies can help.

Aconite   in the early stages, with injection of the conjunctival blood vessels.

Alumina   with dryness.

Apis   in acute cases, with chemosis.

Argentum Nit.   with muco-purulent discharge.

Arsenicum Album   with burning tears – almost a corrosive feeling.

Belladonna   with dilation of the pupils.

Euphrasia   much watering, with burning and with involvement of the edges of the eyelids.

Pulsatilla   conjunctivitis associated with weeping, and much rubbing of the eyes causing inflammation.

Rhus Tox.   for involvement of the eyes in cases of shingles.

Silica   for the conjunctivitis persisting after injury by foreign bodies.

Sulphur   redness of the conjunctivae, not necessarily infected; with hot sensations, worse at night.

CONSTIPATION

In addition to advice on diet and exercise and encouraging a good bowel habit, homoeopathic remedies can be helpful.

Aesculus   when there is a sensation of fullness in the rectum even after a motion.

Alumen   when the stools are very hard and cause bleeding.

Alumina   when there is no urging, but eventually a soft stool with incomplete emptying of the rectum.

Bryonia   when the stools are large, hard and dry, in spite of drinking large quantities of fluids.

Calc. Carb.   when the patient paradoxically feels better when constipated.

Lycopodium   when there are rumblings in the bowels, but no action.

Nitric Acid   with painful defaecation resulting in bleeding, and with the sensation of sharp sticks in the rectum.

Nux Vomica   for sedentary workers with ineffectual urging; even after a motion the rectum never feels empty.

Opium   for 'lazy' bowels with little peristalsis.

Silica   when the stool is low in the rectum but hard to pass.

CONVULSIONS

There is little one can do at the time of a convulsion apart from maintaining the airway and preventing injury, but homoeopathic remedies can be helpful in reducing the recurrence of and the severity of the convulsions.

Aconite   when caused by fright, and during fevers.

Aethusa   with gastroenteritis, especially if there is intolerance of cow's milk.

Belladonna   convulsions during fever, with very flushed face, staring eyes and dilated pupils.

Chamomilla   during teething, especially if accompanied by anger.

Cicuta   with twitchings, jerkings and vertigo.

Cuprum Met.   for convulsions caused by the paroxysms of whooping cough, and with cramps and spasms of fingers.

Glonoine   after too much exposure to the sun.

Ignatia   after punishment and other emotional upsets.

Nux Vomica   convulsions preceded by irritability, and sometimes caused by indigestion.

Zinc Sul.   in infants with pale face and sunken fontanelle.

COUGH

Such a common symptom; but a lot of careful thought is required before it can be treated accurately. If persistent, investigations may be needed to establish a precise diagnosis. The following list of remedies is only a sample of the many which are needed from time to time.

Ammon. Carb.   productive cough, waking the patient in the night.

Antim. Tart.   much rattling in the chest.

Bryonia   with pain in the chest as in pleurisy.

Calc. Carb.   with tickling provoking the cough.

Causticum   dryness, rawness and hoarseness.

Coccus Cacti   with a sensitive throat and paroxysmal cough.

Drosera   paroxysmal cough with laryngitis or laryngeal spasm.

Ipecacuanha   choking cough leading to gagging, nausea and vomiting.

Kali Bich.   with stringy sputum.

Kali Carb.   with lumpy sputum.

Phosphorus   dry racking cough, worse when talking.

Pulsatilla   worse in a warm room, better in the open air.

Rumex   worse on changing from warm air to cold.

Senega   viscid sputum.

Sepia   productive cough at night, but little in the day.

Spongia   paroxysmal dry cough sounding like a bark.

Sticta   dry night cough.

CRAMP

Arnica   for cramps which occur when fatigued.

Calc. Carb.   for patients who are overweight, pale and 'flabby'.

Camphor   for cramps in the calves, with icy coldness of the feet.

Colchicum   for cramps in the soles.

Cuprum Met.   for cramps beginning as twitches.

Nux Vomica   for cramps occurring at night.

Mag. Phos.   for writer's cramp in the fingers.

Veratrum Album   for cramps occurring as a result of diarrhoea and vomiting – similar to cholera.

CROUP

Croup was the popular name for diphtheria, which has now almost been eradicated. But croupy coughs occur quite often, and these remedies should be considered:

Aconite   in the early stages of fevers, especially if brought on by exposure to cold air.

Agaricus   for nervy twitchy children – similar to chorea.

Antim. Tart.   with rattling sounds in the chest as well.

Belladonna   with fever, red face, dry skin and mouth.

Hepar Sul.   when croup develops after midnight.

Ignatia   when the croup has been brought on by fright or other emotion.

Iodum   with wheezing 'sawing' respiration; the child tends to grasp the throat.

Kali Bich.   with tough stringy phlegm.

Lachesis   waking the patient from sleep.

Sambucus   rough sibilant wheezing – and more sweat in the day than when asleep.

Spongia   with a hoarse dry barking cough.

CYSTITIS

True cystitis is due to infection, and antibiotic or chemotherapeutic treatment is usually advisable. When infection is resistant, the homoeopathic nosode of the infecting organism can be expected to cure. At other times, so-called cystitis is an irritation of the bladder and urethra; for example, oxaluria after eating too many strawberries. Advice on hygiene may also be appropriate.

Apis   frequent micturition with sharp stinging pains.

Belladonna   during fever, with concentrated urine.

Benzoic Acid   when the urine smells like a dirty stable.

Berberis   with turbid urine and a slimy mucous sediment.

Cantharis   frequency, and much burning pain.

Causticum   frequency, and dribbling leaking at other times.

Dulcamara   for cystitis due to chilling in cold damp weather.

Lycopodium   when the urine has a deposit of pink urates.

Pulsatilla   when the threshold to pain is low, and slight tension in the bladder provokes micturition.

Sarsaparilla   when pain comes only at the end of micturition.

DANDRUFF

Also known as scurf, and officially as seborrhoea capitis.

Arsenicum Album   very itchy scalp in persons with the typical Arsenicum personality (see Appendix).

Fluoric Acid   dry scaling of the scalp, with marked loss of hair.

Graphites   much scaling of the scalp, often with moistness and crusting, like impetigo.

Mezereum   much itching, and with thick white crusts.

Oleander   a minor remedy, but mentioned by Clarke as having a peculiar symptom – 'biting itching'.

Sepia   moist dandruff.

Sulphur   dandruff provoking much scratching, especially at night.

DEAFNESS

Some of the many forms of deafness, of many different causes, are not amenable to treatment. Some are benefited by surgery, and the persistent catarrhal forms of deafness are particularly suitable for homoeopathic treatment.

Borax   for chronic suppurative otitis media, when antibiotics have not been completely successful.

Causticum   with tinnitus and reverberation of the voice.

China Offic.   for elderly debilitated persons with deafness and much tinnitus.

Kali Mur.   for eustachian catarrhal obstruction.

Lycopodium   with discharge from the ears, and eczema of the outer ear.

Mercurius   has proved valuable in the treatment of 'glue ear'.

Nitric Acid   when hearing is better in noisy surroundings.

Pulsatilla   catarrhal deafness, better in the open air.

Silica   catarrhal deafness with sinusitis as well.

DEBILITY

Every day hundreds of patients tell their doctors they have 'no energy' – usually an understandable exaggeration, really meaning that they have no zest – for many different reasons. Provided that debilitating diseases and psychological factors have been excluded, one of these homoeopathic remedies may restore the strength and enthusiasm required.

Arnica   for those who feel battered and bruised.

Arsenicum Album   weakness, faintness and loss of appetite.

Calc. Carb.   'cold and blue' – cannot get warm enough to get going; like a sluggish engine.

Calc. Phos.   debility after acute illness.

Carbo Veg.   debility after long and exhausting illness.

Kali Carb.   weakness felt mostly in the back, probably signifying the inability to carry one or more burdens.

Kali Phos.   'nervous prostration' – especially in adolescents who are 'burning the candle at both ends' – when the smallest task seems too much to attempt.

Mag. Carb.   tiredness felt mostly in the legs and feet.

Nux Vomica   falls asleep in the early evening, is irritable and dyspeptic.

Sepia   for the person who has lost interest in the family and finds housework exhausting, especially washing-up and laundry.

Silica   when the diet seems adequate, but does not provide the energy one expects.

DELIRIUM

Aconite   worse at night, with much fear.

Agaricus   worse at night and with headache.

Arsenicum Album   worse after midnight and very restless.

Baptisia   disorientated and flushed.

Belladonna   with high fever, dry red skin, and dilated pupils.

Bryonia   with fever, vivid dreams and muttering.

Hyoscyamus   foolish laughter alternating with muttering.

Lachesis   worse at night, very talkative and with tight sensations in the neck and the chest.

Lycopodium   worse from 4 p.m. to 8 p.m., with confusion over words.

Rhus Tox.   with muscle pains and sudden episodes of weeping.

Stramonium   muttering delirium and writhing movements.

Veratrum Album   with much pain.

DELIRIUM TREMENS

This complication of alcoholism usually requires treatment in hospital, but it may be possible to give one of the following remedies as first aid:

Antim. Tart.   for delirium with gastric pain and vomiting with much mucus.

Arsenicum Album   very restless and agitated.

Belladonna   furious delirium with staring eyes.

Hyoscyamus   a quieter delirium, with muttering.

Nux Vomica   with muscle spasms and twitchings.

Stramonium   imagines he (or she) sees animals or insects.

DEPRESSION

This is a complicated subject, especially when one has to consider the extent to which anxiety and other emotions are mixed with depression. Sometimes the cause is obvious and can be dealt with simply; at other times psychiatric advice is necessary. In any case, the homoeopathic remedy can be administered as supplementary aid. Of the many which are valuable, only a few can be mentioned here:

Anacardium   depression, with out-of-character swearing.

Arsenicum Album   restless and self-reproaching.

Aurum Met.   'under a black cloud' and potentially suicidal.

Calc. Carb.   for depression with fears of various kinds.

Ignatia   full of contradictions.

Lilium Tig.   worse in the evenings; tends to throw things about.

Lycopodium   dyspeptic, melancholic and talkative.

Natrum Mur.   weeps in solitude.

Nux Vomica   for depression alternating with bad temper.

Pulsatilla   can't fight against circumstances and doesn't care who sees her weeping.

Staphisagria   easily upset by mere trifles and is resentful.

Sulphur   depressed to the point of 'I don't care'.

DESPAIR

Aurum Met.   for melancholia, when the patient wanders about saying little or nothing, and contemplates suicide.

Calc. Carb.   for indecision, lack of confidence, despair of recovery – and undue sensitivity to cold.

Stannum   when the patient has a sallow face, sunken eyes, is hypochondriacal, and loses hope relatively slowly.

DIARRHOEA

If this is not due to colitis, sprue or other diseases which need investigation and dietary advice, these are some of the remedies which may be helpful:

Arsenicum Album simultaneous diarrhoea and vomiting.

Bryonia due to sour fruit.

Colocynth with much colic, causing the patient to bend double.

Dulcamara after exposure to cold and damp.

Merc. Corr. slimy offensive stools with traces of blood, and with tenesmus.

Natrum Sul. morning diarrhoea, with stools of normal colour, but loose and urgent.

Petroleum worse after cabbage and other green vegetables.

Podophyllum watery yellow stools early in the morning, with a sense of weakness in the rectum.

Pulsatilla worse at night, and variable – no two stools alike.

Sulphur with much offensive flatus, smelling of bad eggs.

DISTENSION OF ABDOMEN

This is a symptom with many causes: some, such as baked beans, quite trivial; others, such as ascites, very serious. If investigations are needed, while waiting for the results, try one of these remedies:

Argentum Nit. with flatulence, and fondness of sugar.

Carbo Veg. wind accumulates in the stomach and is difficult to bring up.

China Offic. fullness in the abdomen, not better for belching.

Lycopodium dyspepsia similar to peptic ulceration, and a feeling of fullness even after only a little food.

Magnesium Phos. distension with colic, or colic with distension.

Millifolium distension due to ascites.

Pulsatilla frequent eructations, and nausea, and compulsion to loosen the clothing.

Raphanus 'incarcerated flatus' which will not move up or down in spite of much rumbling.

Sulphur distension due to flatus which is offensive.

DYSMENORRHOEA (PERIOD PAINS)

If the trouble persists for more than two or three months, it is wise to obtain a doctor's advice before continuing with the chosen remedy.

Actea in stout and red-faced women.

Belladonna worse when lying down; the patient prefers to keep going.

Borax pain radiating down the thighs.

Caulophyllum with much cervical spasm in the first day or night.

Chamomilla angry – 'this is not fair' – 'I can't bear it'.

Cuprum Met. with cramps in the pelvis and in the fingers.

Lachesis worse on waking and worse after taking coffee.

Mag. Phos. with spasmodic pains and cramps, relieved by hot water bottles.

Pulsatilla with a flow of rather dark blood, and when the pain reduces the patient to tears.

Sepia with scanty flow and with dragging sensations in the pelvis.

Viburnum Op. when the periods are delayed and there is much pain, though there is little loss.

DYSPEPSIA (ACUTE)

This section refers to episodes of indigestion of sudden onset, without vomiting or diarrhoea. It will be noticed that three of the remedies appear in both the Acute and the Chronic sections – exemplifying their wide range of use.

Argentum Nit. after eating too much sweet food.

Arsenicum Album burning pain, and desire for frequent small drinks.

Bryonia pressure in the stomach and heavy sensation as if it contained a stone or a weight.

Chamomilla as a result of anger or argument during a meal.

Colocynth griping pains after eating sour fruit.

Nux Vomica due to anxiety and irritability, too much alcohol, after business lunches.

Phosphorus heartburn – even a little water does not stay down long.

Pulsatilla after eating too much fatty food; often better for a walk in the open air.

DYSPEPSIA (CHRONIC)

If indigestion is persistent, it is wise to consider investigation to exclude peptic ulcer and other serious conditions which may need surgery.

Argentum Nit. with eructations of wind and acid – eats too much sugar.

Calc. Carb. especially after fatty and oily food, very fond of boiled eggs, which upset.

Carbo Veg. acidity with much flatulence, in chilly persons who nevertheless like fresh air.

Dioscerea with colic, which is better for straightening or even leaning backwards.

Lycopodium with distension after only a little food, and developing pain which raises suspicion of a peptic ulcer.

Muriatic Acid when there is hyperacidity, especially if lots of antacids have been taken.

Nux Vomica easily upset by many things – alcohol, noise, arguments and so on. Pain occurs typically two hours after food.

Pulsatilla with nausea, leading to vomiting of watery material with mucus.

Robinia constant eructations and vomiting of intensely acid food residue, mostly at night.

Sulphur with regurgitation of food and acid, about one hour after meals; hungry at 11 a.m.

DYSPHAGIA

If painful or difficult swallowing is persistent, investigation will be needed to exclude organic lesions and neurological causes.

China Offic. with much sensitivity – the patient dislikes the throat being touched.

Gelsemium slow difficult swallowing, because the muscles feel weak.

Ignatia globus hystericus – says he or she cannot swallow – but does.

Kali Carb. slow swallowing, with choking.

Lachesis when there is a sense of constriction in the throat and neck (and chest).

Merc. Sol. with slimy mucus, hard to clear and swallow.

Nitric Acid with sharp sticking pains in the throat, as if due to a fish bone.

Phosphorus with burning pain, and traces of blood when the throat is cleared.

Stramonium with dryness of the throat and spasms of the muscles of swallowing.

EARACHE

In selecting the remedy, much depends on the nature of the ache or pain, and on the patient's reaction to it, as well as the cause of the trouble and the modalities. Some of the more important remedies are:

Apis   when there is much swelling of the meatus.

Belladonna   when throbbing is a feature.

Chamomilla   for the child who reacts angrily.

Graphites   when there is much smelly discharge.

Hepar Sul.   when there is pus forming – before it is discharged.

Lachesis   when swallowing markedly increases the pain.

Merc. Sol.   worse at night.

Nitric Acid   for sharp stabbing pains.

Nux Vomica   when the patient is irritable and intolerant of noise.

Pulsatilla   for earache caused by eustachian catarrh.

Sulphur   when the meatus is red and itchy.

ECZEMA

The constitutional remedy is usually needed. Sometimes the causative agent in potency is valuable. In addition, one of the following remedies may be indicated:

Alumina   dry irritating eczema.

Antim. Crud.   eczema of the face and of the genitals.

Bovista   eczema of the back of the hands.

Cicuta   eczema of the chin.

Graphites   eczema of the palms.

Hepar Sul.   moist lesions, very sensitive to the touch.

Kali Sul.   very similar to Pulsatilla – see the Appendix.

Mezereum   eczema of the scalp, with much exudate.

Petroleum   eczema which cracks easily, especially behind the ears.

Radium Brom.   eczema after radiotherapy.

Rhus Tox.   eczema with vesicles

Sulphur   dry, itching and warm.

EUSTACHIAN CATARRH

Asarum   when there are floating sensations, and when there is hypersensitivity to scratching sounds.

Calc. Carb.   when accompanied by enlarged adenoids, and when the constitutional features are present.

Kali Sul.   when there is also yellow nasal catarrh.

Petroleum   when there happens to be some skin disorder, with the cracks or fissures characteristic of Petroleum.

Pulsatilla   the remedy most often needed for Eustachian catarrh, when it is better in the open air – even if the constitutional features are not marked.

EXCITEMENT, AILMENTS AFTER

This section is mainly concerned with children who cannot settle down after parties and other exciting occasions – not illness, but a definite problem in some children.

Capsicum   headache and disturbance of vision.

Coffea   cannot get off to sleep.

Ignatia   as a result of grief, alternate laughter and tears.

Kali Phos.   mainly for adolescents who become overtired from excessive mental and physical exertion.

Nux Vomica   stuttering.

Phosphoric Acid   weakness, and trembling legs.

Pulsatilla   easily excited to tears.

Staphisagria   speechless with excitement, and then stammers.

FAINTING

Ordinary first aid measures are required for any faint; there is seldom time or need to give a homoeopathic remedy. But when faintness persists or recurs:

Aconite   fainting due to fright.

Arnica   after injury.

Arsenicum Album   due to debility, with or without anaemia.

Carbo Veg.   very cold and faint – has been called the 'corpse reviver'; at other times, gasping for air.

Cocculus   as a result of travel sickness.

Hepar Sul.   very sensitive to any pain.

Ignatia   hysterical, and after over-breathing.

Iodum   faint from hunger, when meals are delayed.

Nux Vomica   faint at the sight of blood.

Pulsatilla   fainting in hot stuffy rooms.

FEAR

Experience suggests that homoeopathic remedies for phobias are not mere placebos, but are effective when other measures such as tranquillisers have had little or no positive effect. These are some of the remedies which can be helpful:

Aconite   fear of death; wakes suddenly in fright.

Argentum Nit.   fear causing diarrhoea.

Gelsemium   school phobia.

Kali Carb.   fear of being alone, especially in the evening.

Opium   'petrified' – fear causing a state of helpless inaction.

Phosphorus   fear of the dark, sensitivity to thunder storms, and nightmares.

Pulsatilla   fears leading to floods of tears.

FEET, BURNING

Though this not a formal diagnosis, it is a tiresome symptom, not uncommon, and it is good to be able to offer something in addition to foot baths and foot powders:

Apis   with swelling, and stinging sensations also.

Chamomilla   hot and sweating feet.

Graphites   burning sensations in the soles, worse when walking.

Medorrhinum   also gets cramps and often sleeps in the knee-elbow position.

Phosphorus   burning sensations, especially in the soles, and a tendency to haemorrhages elsewhere.

Pulsatilla   hot sensations in the feet, extending up to the calves, and worse when the feet hang down.

Secale   burning sensations in the hands as well as the feet.

Silica   burning feet at night, and cold clammy feet by day.

Sulphur   burning feet, worse at night – the patient often puts the feet out of bed to cool them.

FRIGHT, EFFECTS OF

Homoeopathic remedies can help as first aid after frightening episodes or situations. They can also help when the reaction persists for days or even weeks.

Aconite   palpitations.

Belladonna   nightmares.

Coffea   insomnia.

Gelsemium   diarrhoea or incontinence, or both.

Hyoscyamus   delirium at night.

Ignatia   hysterical behaviour, including convulsive movements.

Opium   stupor and inaction – 'scared stiff'.

27

GALL BLADDER COLIC

This may need surgical treatment; while investigations are being arranged, one of the following will be helpful:

Berberis   with obstruction, leading to putty-coloured stools and jaundice.

Calc. Carb.   for the classical 'fat, fair and forty' women.

Chelidonium   when the pain radiates in the typical manner to the right scapula.

China Offic.   for pain leading to some degree of shock – with cold clammy skin, chills and rigors.

Colocynth   pain relieved by flexing the back and legs, actually pressing on the painful area.

Dioscerea   better when the back and legs are extended.

Lycopodium   worse between 4 p.m. and 8 p.m.

Mag. Phos.   pain in relatively short spasms, better for heat of hot water bottle.

GINGIVITIS AND PYORRHOEA

It is usually wise to obtain the advice of a dentist.

Arsenicum Album   with a desire for frequent small drinks.

Borax   when there are ulcers on the tongue and cheeks.

Calc. Phos.   swollen, tender and easily bleeding gums.

Carbo Veg.   sore bleeding gums and loose teeth.

Causticum   toothache and ulceration of the gums.

Kali Carb.   with offensive breath.

Merc. Sol.   when the gums are swollen and not close to the teeth; bad breath.

Natrum Mur.   if there is a bitter taste and loose teeth.

Nitric Acid   when there are sharp pains like splinters and when ulceration develops.

Phosphorus   for gums which are soft and 'spongy' and bleed easily.

Silica   when gumboils develop slowly and heal slowly.

GLANDS, ENLARGED LYMPHATIC

The cause of the enlargement must be determined. In addition to any other necessary treatment:

Arum Triphyllum   especially for submaxillary glands.

Barium Carb.   associated with tonsillitis.

Calc. Carb.   when the mediastinal glands are affected and cause cough and other symptoms.

Hepar Sul.   for particularly tender glands, as in the axillae.

Merc. Sol.   if suppuration threatens or occurs.

28   **Silica**   when enlargement is slow and subsidence is also slow.

GLANDULAR FEVER

This infection is an example of the general principle that one does not treat a disease according to its label, but in consideration of its symptoms and signs. Those of glandular fever are: fever, malaise, sore throat, enlarged lymphatic glands, a rash which may look like measles or scarlet fever, tiny points of bleeding in the skin, and sometimes enlargement of the spleen and liver. The selection of the remedy is made according to whichever features of the illness are predominant at the time. Later on the constitutional remedy is usually needed, especially if convalescence is slow.

GOUT

Modern conventional treatment is usually necessary for the acute phases. The homoeopathic constitutional remedy is valuable in the intervals. Various other remedies are worth considering as an addition to control therapy:

Benzoic Acid　when the urine is strongly coloured and smells rather like a stable.

Colchicum　the classical remedy, usually the first to be tried when the constitutional remedy is not obvious.

Ledum　better in cold air and better for cold bathing.

Lycopodium　this is the constitutional remedy most often needed, especially if one foot is hot and the other is cold.

Pulsatilla　when the pains go from one joint to another.

GRINDING OF TEETH

Of course this is not an illness, but it is a tiresome symptom or habit, and potentially harmful to the teeth.

Apis　during fevers, especially if the uvula is swollen.

Belladonna　during fever, with hot red dry skin.

Cicuta　when associated with fits.

Cina　when the child has threadworms, Cina can be given while waiting for the worms to be eliminated.

Podophyllum　when there is intestinal colic as well.

Zincum Met.　when the child is unduly fatigued.

29

HAEMORRHOIDS

Piles usually respond well to **Hamamelis** or **Paeonia** in ointment form. The ointments are equally soothing for internal as well as external piles. When they keep recurring, it is worth considering the use of remedies by mouth.

Aesculus   with backache and prolapse of the rectum.

Aloe   piles 'like grapes', associated with explosive diarrhoea.

Ammon. Carb.   worse during the menses.

Capsicum   with tenesmus and colic.

Causticum   very tender piles.

Collinsonia   also with tenesmus.

Hamamelis   with soreness like a bruise.

Hypericum   very sensitive, and bleeding easily.

Merc. Viv.   with blood and mucus.

Nitric Acid   with pricking sensations and with fissure.

Nux Vomica   with irritability.

Paeonia   much pain during and after bowel action, and often with a fissure.

Pulsatilla   with mucus.

Ruta   with prolapse of the rectum.

Thuja   when the patient also has warts.

Verbascum   with much irritation in the rectum.

HAIR, LOSS OF

Aurum Met.   does not really care if all the hair falls out – is tired of life.

Fluoric Acid   the hair goes dry and brittle and falls out.

Mercurius   with constitutional disturbances – the patient is weak, tremulous and sweaty.

Mezereum   the hair becomes curly and then falls out.

Selenium   the pubic hair falls out as well as the scalp hair.

Sepia   for the patient who is depressed and worried, especially about the family and by the family.

Thallium   with a tendency to conjunctivitis.

HALITOSIS

If the breath remains tainted in spite of advice on oral hygiene and diet:

Aurum Met.   'putrid' breath, especially in girls at puberty.

Chelidonium   when the liver is not working well and the tongue has a thick yellow coat.

Kreasote   with gingivitis, when the gums are inflamed, spongy and bleed easily.

Nitric Acid   with loose teeth, unhealthy gums and the weakness characteristic of all the acids.

Nux Vomica   with sour-smelling breath, due to dyspepsia.

HANDS, DISORDERS OF

Actea   rheumatic pains worse at night.

Apis   acute swelling with much heat.

Argentum Nit.   swelling of the hands, with numbness, especially at the menopause.

Bryonia   swelling of the finger joints, without redness.

Calc. Carb.   cold hands.

Caulophyllum   pains in the wrists and fingers, with stiffness.

Fluoric Acid   constantly moist palms.

Ledum   boring pains in the thumbs, better when cool.

Rhus Tox.   pains in most parts of the hands, especially in the thumbs of persons who do much knitting.

Ruta   sprains of the wrists and fingers.

Sulphur   hot hands.

HAY FEVER

The usual official name, allergic rhinitis, is not a full description because the eyes, the sinuses and the eustachian tubes are so often involved as well. The constitutional remedy is often needed. At other times it is helpful to prescribe the allergen in potency, or a nosode.

Allium Cepa   much lachrymation.

Arsenicum Iod.   dry sneezing and a wheezy chest.

Arundo   much itching in the nostrils.

Dulcamara   worse in the open air.

Euphrasia   burning lachrymation.

Pulsatilla   better in the open air.

Sabsdilla   much itching in the nose, and chest symptoms, 'hay asthma'.

Sanguinaria   hay fever complicated by polypi.

Silica   nasal obstruction, worse on waking and with obstinate sinusitis – in chilly persons.

HEADACHE

No comprehensive list is attempted here; there are so many causes, and so many types. Nevertheless, it is worth presenting a short selection of some of the most useful homoeopathic remedies for headache.

Arnica   after head injury, with or without concussion.

Belladonna   'bursting' headache, with dilated pupils.

Bryonia   better for pressure and keeping still.

Gelsemium   occipital headache and heavy eyelids.

Glonoine   throbbing headache, sometimes due to too much exposure to the sun.

Lachesis   worse on waking, and more on the left side.

Lycopodium   with vertigo, and mainly on the right side.

Magnesium Phos.   neuralgic pain, of a 'shooting, electric' type.

Nux Vomica   the classical remedy for tension headache in the neck.

Pulsatilla   better in the open air and after cold applications.

Sanguinaria   headache gradually worse till noon, then improving.

Spigelia   neuralgic pains, especially in the left temple.

Sulphur   headache worse in the evening.

HEART DISORDERS

Heart failure should receive all necessary conventional treatment. Homoeopathic treatment is often a valuable supplementary measure. For symptoms which are tiresome and uncomfortable but not dangerous, the following remedies are worth remembering:

Apis   relatively sudden pain in the heart with a sense of something like suffocation.

Arnica   when there is a sensation that the heart is being squeezed.

Arsenicum Album   palpitation and some irregularity, with much anxiety and restlessness.

Cactus   the classical homoeopathic remedy for anginal pain, when the chest seems 'in a vice'.

Digitalis   if the pulse is persistently slow, similar to the result of overdosage of digitalis glucosides.

Lachesis   when pain in the heart extends to the neck.

Spigelia   one of the most useful remedies, especially for strong palpitations, detectable by others and sometimes even reported to shake the bed.

HEARTBURN

A quaint word for one kind of dyspepsia, with burning sensations, for which the formal word is pyrosis.

Arsenicum Album if the symptoms are persistent, and associated with debility and loss of weight; investigation is needed.

Capsicum for burning sensations, not only in the stomach, but anywhere in the length of the bowel.

Cicuta when there is throbbing as well as burning.

Colchicum with nausea at the smell, sight or even thought of food.

Lycopodium burning pains with regurgitations or actual vomiting, as in peptic ulceration.

Phosphorus for the patient with burning sensations in the epigastrium and between the shoulder blades.

Sulphur when the symptoms are worse about 11 a.m., with belching as well as burning sensations.

HICCOUGH

Aethusa in infants who cannot tolerate much milk.

Arsenicum Album for hiccoughs associated with carcinoma of the stomach.

Cicuta in infants, especially if there have been convulsions.

Ignatia with other symptoms which are paradoxical and contradictory, raising suspicion of hysteria.

Ipecacuanha with much nausea.

Lycopodium with chronic dyspepsia and hyperacidity.

Mag. Phos. when the patient gets muscle spasms and neuralgic pains elsewhere, for instance cramps in the limbs.

Nux Vomica for hiccoughs occurring an hour or two after food.

Veratrum Viride if hiccoughs follows vomiting.

HYPERACUSIS

Unduly sensitive hearing is not a disease in the ordinary sense, but it is often mentioned as a secondary symptom, and can be useful in deciding the choice of the remedy:

Cannabis Ind. hearing very acute, combined with the exaggeration of duration of time and extent of space.

Coffea excessive sensitivity to music and voices, combined with active and alert thinking, and insomnia.

Nux Vomica the patient's own voice sounds unduly loud to him or her.

Opium undue sensitivity to sounds – an unexpected feature with the classical stupor.

Phosphorus small noises such as the screwing up of paper are 'intolerable', disturbing.

Silica loud noises actually cause pain in the ears.

Tabacum sensitivity to music and loud talking, with tinnitus as well.

HYPOCHONDRIASIS

Undue anxiety about one's health is sometimes an important factor in selecting the remedy.

Actea with depression, like a black cloud over everything.

Arsenicum Album anxiety drives him or her out of bed at night.

Aurum Met. thinks of suicide.

Calc. Carb. fears he or she will go crazy.

Ignatia with a tendency to hysteria.

Natrum Mur. melancholy, tired of life and wants to be alone.

Nux Vomica quarrelsome, and with episodes of violence.

Stannum with weakness, and symptoms predominantly abdominal.

Valerian when there are rapid irrational changes of mood.

HYSTERIA

Actea with gnawing sensations in the epigastrium.

Asafoetida with belchings and sensations of distension.

Crocus has emotional outbursts with quick repentance.

Ignatia with the classical lump in the throat.

Lachesis very talkative.

Moschus with difficult breathing and 'spasms' in the chest.

Platina haughtiness, with contempt.

Tarentula Hisp. with twitching or jerking of muscles.

Valerian excited and sleepless, sometimes with a sensation of floating in the air.

ICTHYOSIS

Dry scaly skin which has less than the normal amount of natural oil in it can predispose to infection, as well as being unsightly and uncomfortable. In combination with suitable creams to soften the skin, one of these remedies can be given by mouth.

Arsenicum Album   dry skin with fine scales, thirsty for small drinks.

Graphites   with cracks in the skin, usually overweight.

Natrum Mur.   dry skin and an itchy patch on the nape of the neck.

Plumbum   very little sweating and usually constipated.

Sepia   with increased pigmentation.

Thuja   for dirty looking skins, with warts.

IMPETIGO

This highly contagious skin disease, characterised by its purulent oozing which forms thick scabs, is usually treated by local antibiotic applications and should be covered to reduce contagion. Homoeopathic remedies are particularly helpful in resistant and recurrent cases.

Antim. Crud.   for impetigo of the nostrils and the corners of the mouth.

Croton Tig.   especially for impetigo of the scrotum.

Graphites   when the oozing and the scabs are honey-coloured.

Hamamelis   also for involvement of the scrotum.

Mezereum   when the scalp is infected and thick crusts form.

Petroleum   with cracks in the skin, especially behind the ears.

IMPOTENCE

Improving the general health by means of the best-indicated homoeopathic remedy may be a valuable factor in dealing with this trouble.

Agnus Castus   ineffectual erection, with general debility and often with absent-mindedness.

Conium   erections not sustained; and associated symptoms in the legs – cramps and coldness.

Graphites   pains in the genitals, interrupting attempts at intercourse; unhealthy skin.

Lycopodium   when it is anticipated that performance will fail; often with chronic dyspepsia.

Sepia   for impotence associated with heaviness and dragging sensations in the genitals.

Sulphur   if there is much itching and redness of the skin in the genital area, sometimes in association with alcoholism.

INFLUENZA

The nosode, **Influenzinum**, is valuable for prophylaxis. The constitutional remedy is valuable for delayed and slow convalescence. In the attack, the following remedies should be remembered:

Aconite in the first few hours of the illness.

Aesculus when the first symptom is backache.

Baptisia for delirium and confusion.

Bryonia when there is chest pain and pleural involvement, as in Bornholm disease.

Camphor when the stage of chill persists.

Eupatorium with pains in the bones.

Gelsemium with chills up and down the spine, and with heavy eyelids.

Glonoine with throbbing headache.

Pyrogen when secondary bacterial infection develops.

Rhus Tox. with muscle pains and stiffness.

Veratrum Album in very severe cases, with delirium, copious sweating, collapse and the rare 'heliotrope' cyanosis.

ITCHING

Agaricus with crawling sensations and sometimes associated with chilblains.

Calc. Carb. better for scratching.

Dolichos very itchy skin but with nothing abnormal to see.

Graphites when the patient scratches till the skin bleeds.

Manganum worse when sweating.

Merc. Sol worse on getting warm.

Mezereum much itching with development of scabs.

Psorinum scratching to the point of bleeding.

Rhus Tox. with urticarial lumps and bumps.

Rumex worse on undressing.

Sulphur worse on getting warm.

Urtica with urticaria, due to many substances in addition to nettles; for reactions to external irritants and to internal allergens.

JAUNDICE

A precise diagnosis is necessary – other treatment may be essential. In addition, one of these remedies may be helpful:

Chelidonium   when there is also gall bladder pain, referred to the tip of the right scapula.

China Offic.   for putty-coloured stools, flatulence and colic.

Crotalus   may be helpful in haemolytic jaundice.

Hydrastis   when the liver is palpably enlarged.

Mercurius   with dull pains in the liver region and a nasty taste in the mouth.

Nux Vomica   for dyspepsia, jaundice, itching skin and associated irritability.

Podophyllum   if gall stones are present, causing obstruction and colic.

KNEES, PAIN IN

When fractures and other conditions which need surgical and other treatment have been excluded:

Apis   for acute synovitis, worse for any form of heat.

Causticum   when the knees cannot be fully extended, with tightness in the hamstrings.

Chamomilla   better, surprisingly, when the joint is fully extended.

Kali Carb.   for dull pains in the knees due to overweight, increasing the strain on the joints.

Ledum   when caused by cold and damp; also after penetrating injuries by stings and by needles.

Natrum Mur.   for prepatellar bursitis – 'housemaid's knee'.

Rhus Tox.   for synovial effusions, with much protective stiffness of the surrounding muscles.

LARYNGITIS

Laryngitis which persists for more than a few days needs investigation. While waiting for the result or, more hopefully, to assist recovery:

Antim. Crud.   for laryngitis due to heat.

Apis   with oedema of the uvula and dysphagia as well.

Arnica   after much shouting or other over-use of the voice.

Arum   for laryngitis of singers, preachers and other public speakers.

Barium Carb.   for simple chronic laryngitis.

Carbo Veg.   for weakness of voice in old people.

Hepar Sul.   in the later stages of bronchitis with laryngitis, when the cough has loosened but the hoarseness persists.

Lachesis   for chronic laryngeal strain in very talkative people.

Phosphorus   with irritating dryness of the throat and larynx, and sometimes specks of blood with the phlegm.

Rhus Tox.   the voice improves with continued talking.

Spongia   laryngitis with an associated dry 'barking' cough.

LEUCORRHOEA

If there is reason to suspect that there is infection which may have been acquired sexually, the disease is notifiable and should receive conventional treatment. In other cases, homoeopathic remedies should be considered, with special reference to constitutional features.

Alumina   with raised itchy spots in the vagina.

Borax   when the discharge is clear, like egg-white.

Carbo An.   if the discharge burns the skin and stains the clothing yellow.

Kreasote   yellow offensive discharge, causing itching and burning.

Medorrhinum   for symptoms remaining after treatment of gonorrhoea.

Pulsatilla   when the discharge is mucoid, rather like nasal mucus.

Sepia   useful for prepubertal leucorrhoea, and also for cases in adults when there is much dragging sensation in the pelvic organs.

LIMBS: FIDGETY, JERKY OR RESTLESS

Fidgeting can be embarrassing; jerking, especially just when the patient is going to sleep, can be very annoying; and restlessness is often a valuable pointer to the similimum.

Fidgeting   Kali Bich., Phosphorus or Zincum.

Jerking when going to sleep   Agaricus, Belladonna, Ignatia, Kali Carb., Sepia.

Jerking as a result of sudden noise   Borax, Carbo Veg., Opium.

General restlessness   Arsenicum Album, Calc. Phos., Hyoscyamus, Pulsatilla, Stramonium, Tarentula.

LUMBAGO

Aconite   as a result of exposure to draughts.

Arnica   as a result of injury or when the muscles feel bruised.

Bellis Perennis   worse after stooping in the open air, typically after gardening.

Berberis   worse on waking.

Bryonia   worse on any movement and markedly relieved by staying still.

Dulcamara   worse after much stooping and exposure to cold and damp.

Nux Vomica   after getting chilled.

Rhododendron   worse when a storm is approaching.

Rhus Tox.   when stiffness is a most marked feature and is gradually relieved by continued gentle motion.

MEASLES

This is a less serious problem nowadays, but cases still occur, and prompt treatment reduces the risk of complications.

Aconite   in the early stages when frequent cough prevents sleep.

Belladonna   for the child with very red face, headache, sore throat, before the sweating develops.

Bryonia   when the rash is slow to appear.

Euphrasia   if conjunctivitis is a prominent feature.

Kali Bich.   when the cough produces stringy sputum and the voice is hoarse.

Mercurius   when excess catarrh persists.

Pulsatilla   for the child who is very sorry for himself or herself, with copious catarrh, and dislikes heavy bedclothes.

Sulphur   if the rash is dusky and slow to clear.

The nosode, **Morbillinum**, is valuable for prophylaxis, and also for sequelae of measles, when the patient has never been really well since the infection.

MEMORY, IMPAIRED

It would be rash to claim that homoeopathic treatment would improve the memory, but the complaint of poor memory is a valuable clue to selecting the remedy for other disorders.

Aethusa   poor memory and poor concentration.

Anacardium   tends to swear because of the frustration caused by poor memory.

Barium Carb.   absent-minded and inattentive.

Cocculus   slow in remembering and easily distracted.

Lycopodium   thinks his memory is worse than it really is.

Plumbum   forgets words and is slow to grasp ideas.

Rhododendron   thoughts disappear while they are being put into words.

Sulphur   poor memory, especially for names.

MENOPAUSE, DISORDERS OF

Aurum Met.   hot flushes and melancholia.

Glonoine   throbbing in the head, with flushing.

Graphites   flushing, especially of the face, sometimes with nose-bleeds and a tendency to put on weight.

Kali Carb.   loss of appetite, regurgitations and backache.

Lachesis   flushes, a sense of constriction round the neck, talkative; all symptoms worse on waking.

Sepia   hot sweats, backache, especially in the sacral area, with sinking or dragging sensations.

Sulphuric Acid   flushes worse in the evenings and after exertion; general weariness.

MENORRHAGIA

The cause of heavy periods should always be determined. While waiting for investigations:

Belladonna   loss of bright red blood, in red-faced women.

Borax   when the periods are early and profuse, with colic and nausea.

Bovista   if the flow is worse at night.

Calc. Carb.   for women who are pale, overweight and chilly.

Chamomilla   with clots, and intolerance of pain.

China Offic.   when the clots are dark.

Ferrum Met.   better when walking about slowly.

Ipecacuanha   bright loss, with nausea.

Phosphorus   no clots and restless, fidgety.

Sabina   intermittent loss.

Secale   thin watery loss, with no clots.

Sepia   with bearing down pains and a tendency to prolapse.

MENTAL EXHAUSTION (BRAIN FAG)

Aethusa   distracted and exhausted by too much mental work of different kinds in rapid succession – confused.

Anacardium   loss of memory or fear of loss, especially before exams.

Calc. Phos.   after much worry or illness.

Gelsemium   during or after influenza.

Kali Phos.   in adolescence.

Lycopodium   with confusion in choosing the right words.

Phosphoric Acid   with physical weakness as well.

Picric Acid   with indifference, little will power and persistent headache.

Silica   with impaired memory due to overwork and with headaches, usually in the sinuses.

Zinc Met.   with poor memory, after insufficient sleep, trembling and fidgeting.

MOUTH ULCERS AND VESICLES

Borax   mouth ulcers with grey bases, very sore.

Hepar Sul.   very sensitive vesicles, proceeding to ulceration with yellow base; gingivitis too.

Merc. Corr.   ulcers, excess saliva and a bad taste.

Natrum Mur.   Blisters like pearls.

MUMPS

In addition to the usual management and nursing required for the acute phase, homoeopathic remedies are helpful. The nosode, **Parotidinum**, is valuable when convalescence is slow.

Aconite   in the early febrile stage.

Calc. Carb.   for pale fat children.

Chamomilla   when there is bad temper and intolerance.

Jaborandi   this contains various alkaloids, including Pilocarpine, and is almost specific for mumps.

Phytolacca   if there are neck symptoms and sore throat as well as the swelling of the parotid glands.

Pulsatilla   if the testes become involved and orchitis develops.

MUSCLE PAINS

Aconite   for stiff neck, especially if due to a draught of air.

Arnica   for bruised muscles.

Bryonia   for pain in the intercostal muscles, with or without involvement of the pleura.

Causticum   for pain in the hamstrings, with limited extension.

Dulcamara   for aching muscles due to cold damp conditions.

Ledum   for muscles involved in stab wounds and hypodermic injections.

Nux Vomica   for pain in the muscles at the back of the neck, associated with tension headaches.

Phytolacca   for muscle pains in heavily built persons; especially for pain in the deltoids.

Rhus Tox.   for painful stiff muscles.

NAILS, DISORDERS OF

Alumina   for brittle and spotted nails.

Antim. Crud.   for horny thick nails, especially toenails.

Arsenicum Album   when the nails crack easily.

Calc. Carb.   for soft nails which break off easily.

Graphites   when the nails grow thick and distorted.

Secale   when the nails separate easily from their beds.

Silica   for brittle and yellow nails.

Thuja   when the nails are brittle and when the patient also has condylomata or warts.

NAUSEA

A common symptom with many causes, and for which there are many homoeopathic remedies. The cause should be established before treatment is begun. These are some of the remedies most often used:

Arsenicum Album   worse after midnight.

Calc. Carb.   worse after drinking milk and in the morning.

Cocculus   especially for travel nausea and sickness.

Colchicum   very sensitive to the smell of cooking.

Ipecacuanha   for persistent nausea, with headache as well.

Iris   one of the remedies for migraine, when nausea is a pronounced feature.

Kali Carb.   as a result of excitement and of motion.

Lobelia   when there is much salivation with the nausea.

Nux Vomica   worse in the morning, as with a 'hangover'.

Pulsatilla   for nausea during pregnancy, better in the open air, often accompanied by much catarrh.

Tabacum   better in the open air, away from tobacco smoke.

NECK, STIFFNESS OF

Aconite   for acute torticollis due to draughts of cold air.

Calc. Carb.   with hoarseness and enlarged neck glands.

Cicuta   when the neck is stiff and turned to one side.

Dulcamara   stiffness after a chill, better for hot applications.

Mag. Phos.   sudden stiffness with neuralgic pains.

Nux Vomica   for tension in the back of the neck, with tension headache and irritability.

Phytolacca   stiffness due to sore throat, tonsillitis, quinsy, in muscular persons with 'bull neck'.

Rhus Tox.   when the stiffness extends to the trapezius.

NEURALGIA

Aconite   for facial neuralgia caused by cold draughts.

Arsenicum Album   for intermittent burning neuralgic pains.

Chelidonium   for intercostal neuralgia, worse from touch as well as worse from motion.

Colocynth   for trigeminal neuralgia, especially if the pain has a 'tearing' quality.

Kalmia   for neuralgia in the right side of the face and in the right arm.

Mag. Phos.   for paroxysmal pains like electric shocks in the limbs, especially in the sciatic plexus.

Ranunculus Bulb.   for intercostal and supraorbital neuralgias.

Spigelia   for sudden sharp pains in the left temple, often with associated palpitations.

NOSE, DISEASES OF

This section is mainly concerned with bleeding from the nose. See also the sections on Catarrh and Sinusitis.

Arnica   for bruising and bleeding after injury.

Belladonna   red face, throbbing headache and bleeding.

Calc. Carb.   when there are polypi with associated catarrh and obstruction.

Carbo Veg.   for old people who sneeze a lot and then get nose-bleeds.

Ferrum Phos.   especially for children whose noses bleed during feverish illnesses.

Hamamelis   when nose-bleeds are frequent, and when there is engorgement of veins elsewhere, as in the legs.

Phosphorus   frequent and profuse sudden nose-bleeds.

Pulsatilla   polypi causing nasal obstruction.

Sanguinaria   polypi, much sneezing and headaches.

Sulphur   itching nose, causing much sneezing.

NUMBNESS

If numbness persists, a neurological assessment is needed.

Aconite   numbness and tingling of the hands and feet as in the hyperventilation syndrome.

Chamomilla   numbness of the hands, worse when grasping.

Conium   numbness of the legs, beginning in the feet and working upwards.

Ignatia   numbness of the heels, worse when walking.

Natrum Mur,   numbness, tingling and exhaustion.

Phosphorus   burnings and tinglings as well as numbness.

Secale   numbness, coldness and threat of gangrene.

OBESITY

The essential treatment of obesity is, of course, advice on diet, habits and exercise. Obesity or the tendency to it is a valuable clue for finding the constitutional remedy for other disorders.

Calc. Carb.   with enlarged glands.

Capsicum   'lax, lazy, fat and red' – with burning sensations anywhere in the alimentary system.

Ferrum   red-faced and subject to dyspepsia.

Graphites   with a tendency to skin diseases.

Hepar Sul.   hypersensitive and liable to develop recurrent small boils.

Kali Carb.   with backache and catarrhal tendencies.

OVARIES, DISORDERS OF

Actea   ovarian pains at puberty.

Apis   ovarian tenderness, especially on the left.

Colocynth   ovarian neuralgia, associated with intestinal colic.

Hepar Sul.   tenderness of the ovaries, part of a general hypersensitivity.

Lachesis   pain mainly on the left, worse for tight clothing.

Lilium Tig.   right ovarian pain, extending to the thighs.

PANIC

Aconite   at night, on waking after bad dreams, during fever.

Argentum Nit.   stage fright and exam 'funk'.

Arsenicum Album   when alone.

Gelsemium   shaking with fright.

Opium   'paralysed' by fright, unable to act.

Stramonium   excessive fear of the dark.

PERSPIRATION AND BODY ODOUR

Arsenicum Album   sweaty palms, worse in company.

Calc. Carb.   sweating, especially of the head, in infancy.

China Offic.   sweating and debility after illness.

Fluoric Acid   the sweat has a sour smell.

Merc. Sol.   when the sweat has an offensive odour.

Phosphorus   exhausting sweats, especially at night.

Psorinum   persistent bad odour in spite of washing.

Sepia   excessive sweating, especially menopausal.

Silica   cold sweaty feet.

Sulphur   hot sweaty feet.

PHARYNGITIS

Apis   with swelling of the uvula – can hardly swallow.

Belladonna   when the pharynx is hot, dry and red.

Capsicum   if there is a hot smarting sensation, as if caused by pepper.

Kali Bich.   with the sensation of a hair stuck in the throat.

Lac Caninum   when the soreness goes from one side to the other.

Lachesis   if there is a bluish tinge of the pharynx, a sense of constriction, and dysphagia.

Merc. Cyan.   when there is a grey exudate.

Merc. Sol.   with much saliva and retching.

Nitric Acid   if there are pricking sensations, as from a fish bone.

Phytolacca   when there is a feeling of a hot lump in the throat, and swallowing causes pain which radiates to the ears.

PHLEBITIS

The risk of fragments of thrombus breaking off and causing embolism should always be remembered and guarded against. In addition to such measures, one of these remedies may be helpful:

Apis   in the early stages, with pain, redness and swelling.

Arnica   when the phlebitis is the result of known injury.

Fluoric Acid   if there are hard 'knots' in the affected veins.

Hamamelis   when the pain and tenderness is sufficient to cause lameness.

Hepar Sul.   for marked sensitivity – when the patient can hardly bear any touching of the area.

Lachesis   when there is a purple tinge of the affected area.

Vipera   if there is a bursting sensation in the limb and if it is much worse when allowed to hang down.

PLEURAL PAIN

This title is chosen so as to include pain with or without fever or effusion – a broader collection of disorders – not just pleurisy in the usual sense.

Belladonna   in the early stages of acute febrile pleurisy.

Bryonia   the remedy most often needed for sharp pleural pains, better when lying still on the painful side.

Chelidonium   when there is much coughing, with pain behind the sternum, referred from the mediastinum.

Hepar Sul.   useful in later stages, when recovery is slow, and the chest is sensitive to cold air.

Natrum Sul.   for pleural pain accompanied by dry cough, worse at night, better sitting up and pressing on the painful area.

Rumex   when the pain is accompanied by tickling and raw sensation in the trachea.

Sticta   for the patient who starts coughing and finds it very difficult to stop.

POLYPI, NASAL

Cadmium Sul.   with a sense of tightness at the root of the nose.

Calc. Carb.   with loss of sense of smell, and sometimes with swelling of the upper lip.

Phosphorus   the polypi bleed easily when the nose is blown.

Psorinum   with chronic post-nasal drip, especially in patients who tend to be chilly.

Pulsatilla   with plentiful catarrh.

Thuja   the remedy most often indicated for warts and other kinds of lumps on the skin, as well as for nasal polypi.

47

PREMENSTRUAL TENSION

Calc. Carb.   tenderness of the breasts.

Causticum   pessimistic and irritable.

Conium   with sore breasts and cold legs.

Graphites   distinct increase in weight.

Kreasote   restless and irritable.

Lachesis   when there is fluid retention and heaviness of the breasts.

Lycopodium   cross and melancholic.

Natrum Mur.   also for fluid retention; irritable and sad.

Nux Vomica   very irritable and quarrelsome.

Pulsatilla   weepy and with painful breasts.

Sepia   depressed, irritable and with reduced libido.

PROSTATE, ENLARGEMENT OF

Eventually, surgery may be needed, but homoeopathic remedies may delay or even avoid the need for surgery.

Barium Carb.   especially for thin under-weight persons, with frequency and a slow stream.

Calc. Carb.   for heavy, sluggish and apprehensive men, when the prostate produces much mucus.

Conium   when frequency is especially troublesome at night and worse after any alcohol.

Iodum   if the gland is hard – and arouses suspicion of carcinoma, needing investigation.

Pulsatilla   with itching and oozing of mucus from the meatus.

Sabal   when there are stinging pains on micturition, and the bladder and urethra seem unduly irritable.

PRURITUS VULVAE

This tiresome, distressing and sometimes embarrassing complaint may be due to infection, and then will need appropriate conventional treatment. If there is no discharge:

Ambra   itching worse at night.

Merc. Sol.   much burning after scratching, and worse when wetted by urine.

Nitric Acid   with pricking like needles, worse while walking.

Petroleum   with visible dermatitis of the vulva.

Platinum   with voluptuous crawling sensations.

Rhus Tox.   when there are small vesicles and these are sometimes the manifestation of herpes.

Sepia   in slim brunettes, especially during pregnancy.

PSORIASIS

This is a constitutional disturbance of the skin, and needs a careful assessment of the whole person. The family history as well as the personal history are important.

Arsenicum Album   see the Appendix on Constitutional Remedies.

Cicuta Vir.   thick crusts with much burning and itching.

Clematis   when pustules form in or under the scaly patches.

Graphites   with thick gummy exudate indicating infection.

Kali Ars.   if the itching is worse in the warm, and especially if there is more scaling than usual.

Petroleum   when there is a history of use of ointments with a paraffin base.

Psorinum   when the skin never seems really clean.

Sulphur   see the Appendix.

RHEUMATISM

This section concerns the muscles, not the joints.

Arnica   worse after bruising and over-exertion.

Bryonia   worse for movement, better for rest and pressure.

Causticum   better in damp weather; when there is a tendency to contracture, especially of the hamstrings.

Colchicum   worse at night and in winter.

Dulcamara   when caused by or aggravated by cold and damp.

Kali Iod.   when the muscle pains are tearing or darting.

Ledum   for muscle pains after stings, puncture wounds and injections.

Merc. Sol.   worse at night and often with 'sour' sweat.

Pulsatilla   for muscle pains which shift from place to place.

Rhus Tox.   with much stiffness, especially of the hands and fingers; worse on starting to move, but soon better on continued movement.

Ruta   for pains in tendons as well as in muscles.

SACRAL AND SACRO-ILIAC PAIN

Appropriate movements, exercises and manipulations are usually effective.

Aesculus sacro-iliac pain, worse when walking slowly or standing.

Agaricus with sensations of bruising, pressure or weight.

Aloe sacral pains accompanying diarrhoea and piles.

Berberis pain referred from the rectum.

Rhus Tox. when the pain results in marked stiffness – almost immobility.

Sepia with dragging sensations in the pelvis.

Sulphur when the pain extends to the groins.

Tellurium for pains shooting up from the sacrum and down to the thighs.

SALIVATION

Excess or deficiency of saliva is obviously not a disease, but can be a useful clue in helping to find the right remedy for other disorders.

Excess

Allium after eating – paradoxical.

Ipecacuanha with nausea and gagging as a result of coughing.

Iris with migraine or similar headache.

Merc. Sol. with sore gums – worse at night.

Nitric Acid with mouth ulcers and prickings.

Veratrum Album with cold sweat and faintness.

Deficiency

Arsenicum Album when the mouth is dry with fear.

Barium Carb. with numbness as well as dryness.

Belladonna when the mouth is hot and dry.

Bryonia little saliva, but little thirst.

Capsicum with burning sensations and dryness.

Carbo Veg. when the tongue is rough as well as dry.

Hyoscyamus in low muttering delirium.

Natrum Sul. if the tongue looks and feels slimy but dry.

Nux Moschata when there is so little saliva that the tongue sticks to the palate.

Silica if the mouth and tongue are dry in spite of a fair amount of thin saliva.

SCIATICA

Ammon. Mur. worse when sitting and the hamstrings feel short.

Arsenicum Album especially for older people.

Colocynth worse because of cold and damp.

Dioscerea better when the spine is extended.

Gelsemium worse when resting at night.

Kali Carb. when sciatic pain is made worse by coughing, especially about 3 a.m.

Lycopodium worse in the afternoon and when lying on the affected side.

Mag. Phos. for the classical 'electric' shooting pains down the leg, worse on coughing and better for flexion of the spine.

SCREAMING AND CRYING CHILDREN

First it is necessary to determine if there is any physical cause for screaming which requires treatment. These remedies are useful when there is a habit of apparently unnecessary screaming.

Antim. Tart. for crying, whining and frequent waking.

Belladonna during fever and delirium, and as a result of nightmares.

Calc. Carb. for the child who cries in his or her sleep.

Chamomilla cries angrily till picked up.

Cicuta when screaming leads to howling, then moaning, then weeping.

Cina for noisy delirium and dislike of even being looked at.

Phosphorus when nightmares cause screaming, especially in dark haired children.

Pulsatilla more for pitiful weeping, especially in fair haired children.

SHIVERING, CHILLS AND RIGORS

Aconite with fever.

Arsenicum Album with waves of icy coldness.

Astacus with urticaria due to shell fish.

Bellis Perennis as a result of having a cold drink when over-heated.

Camphor for the patient who asks alternately for warmth and then for cold air.

Carbo Veg. despite the shivering, wants the window opened so that he or she can sit in a draught.

Cinchona when fever and sweating is preceded by rigors.

SINUSITIS

Persistent or recurrent sinusitis, not responding well to other treatments, is often improved by the well-indicated homoeopathic remedy.

Agaricus   when sinusitis causes widespread headaches.

Belladonna   when there is pain, especially in the frontal sinuses, worse on stooping.

Graphites   if blowing the nose leaves fairly prolonged pain.

Hepar Sul.   when the catarrh is yellow and the face is hypersensitive.

Kali Bich.   when the catarrh is stringy.

Kali Carb.   when the catarrh is lumpy.

Pulsatilla   when nasal obstruction is variable and causes pain above the eyes.

Silica   when the pain feels as if it is in the bones surrounding the sinuses

Spigelia   for sinusitis with neuralgic type of pain.

SKIN, CRACKS AND FISSURES IN

Alumina   for the hard dry skin of old people, easily cracked — especially the hands.

Calc. Carb.   when the skin cracks in the winter.

Graphites   for cracks in the nostrils, on the lips, behind the ears, and of the nipples.

Nitric Acid   when cracks bleed easily, and for cracks with crusts forming on the edges of the nostrils.

Natrum Mur.   especially for cracks in the centre of the lower lip.

Petroleum   for cracks in the skin of the palms and behind the ears, worse in winter.

Sarsaparilla   for cracks in the skin of the feet, and of the hands, fingers and thumbs, and at the corners of the mouth.

Sepia   'the washerwoman's remedy' — for cracks resulting from prolonged immersion in water.

Sulphur   for intertrigo — cracks or splits in the skin folds, when the skin is softened, macerated, and often infected.

SLEEP, DISTURBANCES OF

Aconite very restless sleep, twisting and turning and undoing the bedclothes.

Arnica unable to sleep because overtired, and the bed feels hard.

Belladonna when the limbs jerk just as the patient is getting off to sleep; also for nightmares.

Calc. Carb. for the child who cries or moans in sleep; also when there is marked sweating of the head during sleep.

Coffea kept awake by continuing thoughts: 'Can't switch off'.

Ignatia yawns a lot but can't get off to sleep.

Kali Carb. wakes about 3 a.m. and can't get back to sleep.

Nux Vomica insomnia because of dyspepsia, eventually sleeps, but wakes with a 'hangover' or something very like it.

Opium deep sleep lasting longer than normal, hard to rouse.

Phosphorus when there are frequent nightmares.

Sambucus wakes gasping for breath, as if suffocating.

Spigelia kept awake by palpitations, which are sometimes strong enough to disturb the partner.

Sulphur needs an extra pillow to reduce a sense of congestion in the head; the limbs get unpleasantly hot, and the patient sticks them out of bed.

SMELL; SENSE OF SMELL DIMINISHED

It would be rash to claim that homoeopathic remedies can alone restore the full sense of smell, but when catarrh is obviously a factor in the problem, they are likely to be helpful.

Anacardium when there is nasal obstruction.

Calc. Carb. when polyps are present.

Hepar Sul. when there is yellow catarrh, a tendency to sweating and an improvement in warm weather.

Influenzinum as a consequence of influenza.

Phosphorus with burning sensations and a tendency to nosebleeds.

Pulsatilla when the amount of catarrh varies markedly from hour to hour, and is better in the open air.

Sepia with dryness of the nasal passages.

Silica when there is associated sinusitis.

SPRAINS

Arnica   for sprains involving the wrist or ankle, especially when there is a haematoma.

Calc. Phos.   for sprains of the carpus.

Rhus Tox.   for sprains in rheumatic subjects, with much stiffness and reluctance to move.

Ruta   for most sprains – almost a specific.

STAMMERING

The essential treatment of stammering and stuttering is speech therapy, to encourage good breathing and good phonation. But homoeopathic remedies can be helpful as well.

Belladonna   especially for children who talk too fast.

Causticum   when stammering is accompanied by grimacing.

Merc. Sol.   with tremors, especially of the tongue.

Nux Vomica   for the patient who is 'jumpy' and irritable, and tends to omit or transpose syllables as well as stammering.

Stramonium   when there are exaggerated movements of the limbs while talking.

STIFFNESS OF MUSCLES AND OF JOINTS

Apis   for stiffness due to synovitis.

Arnica   for stiffness after exertion and strenuous games.

Bryonia   stiffness of elbows and knees, better when quite still.

Calc. Sul.   when the stiffness is in the shoulders.

Causticum   stiffness around the knees and ankles, with tightness of the hamstrings, preventing full extension of the knees.

Chelidonium   when the legs are stiff, heavy and lame.

Ledum   for stiffness due to cold and damp.

Rhus Tox.   for stiffness which is worse on first movement, improving during continued movement, especially in the wrists, hands, fingers and thumbs.

Silica   for stiffness associated with scars.

STROKES

The old name apoplexy is best avoided. The relatively new term, CVA, cerebral vascular accident, is not really appropriate because a stroke is not an accident, but a lesion. Hospitals are often reluctant to admit patients with strokes until they have survived the first forty-eight hours. Meanwhile, homoeopathy can help.

Arnica   often chosen because the cerebral lesion is similar to a bruise, a haematoma.

Belladonna   when the face is flushed and there is throbbing headache.

Natrum Mur.   when the face is pale and there is throbbing headache.

Nux Vomica   when the stroke occurs after a heavy meal or too much alcoholic drink.

Opium   when the patient is unconscious, breathing heavily, and the face is dusky or cyanosed.

Sulphur   for the heavy red-faced beer-drinking type.

Veratrum Album   when the clinical picture is one of 'collapse' – shocked, sweating and cold.

STYES

Graphites   when the styes produce much sticky honey-coloured exudate, as occurs with impetigo.

Phosphorus   when there is twitching of the eyelids, and a burning sensation in them.

Pulsatilla   when the eyelids are stuck together on waking.

Staphisagria   when there is frontal headache.

Staphylococcinum   when infection with staphylococci is proved, or suspected, and styes persist, this nosode can be expected to stimulate the development of better resistance to the germs.

Thuja   Hahnemann's chief antipsoric remedy.

SUNSTROKE

This is a convenient term to include the ill-effects of over-exposure to the sun, and also the ill-effects of other forms of heat.

Aconite   with fever, confusion and apparent stupidity.

Antim. Crud.   after too much exertion in the sun.

Belladonna   with throbbing headache, hot dry skin and dilated pupils.

Cuprum Met.   when much sweating has caused excess salt loss and cramps.

Gelsemium   with giddiness, as if intoxicated.

Glonoine   with throbbing headache, flushed face and sweating.

Natrum Mur.   when the patient is irritable and hates any fuss.

55

SYNOVITIS

Effusion into a joint often causes some instability. This applies especially to the knee, and it is usually wise to support the knee with a crêpe type of bandage.

Apis   in the early stages, when the joint is painful, hot and swollen.

Arnica   when there is evidence or suspicion of bleeding into the joint.

Belladonna   when the pain is eased by hot applications.

Bryonia   especially for synovitis of small joints.

Causticum   for subacute or chronic synovitis, with associated weakness of the joint.

Colchicum   for acute synovitis, especially of the legs, with hot tearing pains, like gout.

Pulsatilla   for hot swellings, especially of the elbow and of the knee, with the swelling visible above the patella.

Rhus Tox.   for effusion and stiffness of the surrounding muscles.

Ruta   for traumatic synovitis associated with sprains.

TEETHING TROUBLES

Actea   when nervous and restless during teething.

Borax   for teething complicated by aphthous or ulcerative stomatitis; and when there is dislike of downward motion, when being put into the cot.

Calc. Carb.   when teething is late, and associated with diarrhoea and green stools.

Calc. Phos.   for babies who are late in teething, late in sitting up and late in walking.

Chamomilla   fretful and angry – yells till picked up and is quiet until put back in the cot.

Kreasote   when the teeth have poor enamel which begins to decay soon after eruption.

Merc. Sol.   when there is excess salivation during teething, sore gums and diarrhoea.

TEMPERAMENT AND MOOD

The constitutional temperament and the mood of the moment can be useful guides to the correct remedy for psychological disturbances and for many disorders with a predominantly somatic manifestation. Homoeopathic remedies are often valuable alternatives to conventional tranquillisers, antidepressives and anxiolytics.

This list shows only one remedy for each temperament or mood, leaving room for the reader to make additions as required.

Angry   Chamomilla.

Apathetic   Phosphoric Acid.

Company wanted   Phosphorus.

Company shunned   Natrum Mur.

Complacent   Arnica.

Confused   Baptisia.

Despairing   Aurum.

Excitable   Belladonna.

Frightened   Aconite.

Haughty   Platinum.

Humble   Pulsatilla.

Hurried   Lilium Tig.

Hysterical   Ignatia.

Impatient   Sulphur.

Indifferent   Sepia.

Irritable   Nux Vomica.

Lamenting   Lycopodium.

Lazy   Calc. Carb.

Obstinate   Tub. Bov.

Quarrelsome   Petroleum.

Raging   Hyoscyamus.

Resentful   Staphisagria.

Restless   Arsenicum Album.

Sad   Stannum.

Taciturn   Silica.

Talkative   Lachesis.

TESTES, DISORDERS OF

Arnica   after injury and bruising.

Aurum Met.   chronic neuralgic pain, causing depression.

Belladonna   acute 'intolerable' pain.

Clematis   persistent chronic pains extending to the groins and the thighs.

Hamamelis   when the testes are very sensitive, and when the skin of the scrotum is disordered.

Pulsatilla   acute pain with much swelling, as in mumps.

Rhododendron   aching in the testes, worse before thunderstorms.

Spongia   persistent aching due to much coughing.

THIRST, ABNORMAL

When diabetes (mellitus or insipidus) have been excluded, consider:

Arsenicum Album   wants to drink little and often.

Belladonna   when the mouth is hot, dry and red.

Bryonia   for thirst for large quantities.

Dulcamara   wants hot drinks, but they are vomited.

Phosphorus   thirsty for cold drinks, which are soon vomited.

Stramonium   wants sour drinks such as lemon juice.

Sulphur   is thirsty but not hungry.

THRUSH (APHTHOUS STOMATITIS)

Antim. Tart.   for children, especially when they vomit milk.

Arsenicum Album   marasmic cases, with ulcers and prostration and low fever, especially if there is simultaneous vomiting and diarrhoea.

Borax   for simple stomatitis, with established ulcers – the old-fashioned Borax in Glycerine was unwitting, or unacknowledged, homoeopathy.

Capsicum   with hot sensations in the mouth, made worse by cold water.

Kali Chlor.   with salivation and tenderness of the salivary glands.

Merc. Sol.   with salivation and slimy diarrhoea.

Natrum Mur.   with herpetic vesicles on the lips.

TINNITUS

Noises in the head or in the ears of a purely subjective origin are usually resistant to treatment, and it is rash to hold out hopes of a cure. Sometimes the well-chosen remedy can bring some relief:

China Offic.   for tinnitus associated with deafness, and sometimes with headache and vertigo.

Graphites   for tinnitus associated with the so-called 'boilermaker's deafness' – when the hearing is better in a noise.

Lachesis   when the noises are most pronounced on waking.

Petroleum   for noises of a whizzing nature, as of a breeze.

Phosphoric Acid   for tinnitus associated with debility, weakness and vertigo.

Pulsatilla   when the noises are worse when there is upper respiratory catarrh.

Spigelia   for tinnitus with neuralgic pains in the ears, intermittent rather than continuous.

Sulphur   when the noises are worse at night.

TONGUE, DISORDERS OF

The tongue is abnormal in many diseases – in some anaemias and as a result of various infections. The possibility of malignant changes must be remembered.

Aconite tingling or numb.

Antim. Crud. lumpy and tender – in old people who do not feel the cold.

Apis swollen and redder than usual – often associated with oedema of the uvula.

Arsenicum Album with a sore red tip.

Arum cracked and bleeding.

Belladonna dry and reddened.

Bryonia dry and pale, even nearly white.

Cantharis scalded or burned.

Hydrastis burned, raw and with prominent taste buds.

Merc. Sol. swollen, slimy or moist, and indented by the teeth.

Natrum Mur. patterned – sometimes called 'geographical'.

Rhus Tox. with a sore red tip – especially if there is pain, stiffness and cracking in the jaw joints.

TONSILLITIS

Acute attacks of tonsillitis may need antibiotics. Chronic or recurrent tonsillitis usually responds well to homoeopathy.

Barium Carb. for undersized children with recurrent attacks.

Calc. Carb. for fat chilly children with a tendency to persistent enlargement of the cervical glands.

Hepar Sul. with much inflammation and yellow exudate, when the soreness is better for warm drinks.

Lachesis with marked dislike of anything touching the throat, causing a sense of constriction.

Lycopodium also with a sense of constriction and when the symptoms are worse about 4 p.m. to 8 p.m.

Merc. Sol. when there is marked sweating, bad breath and extra salivation.

Nitric Acid with much exudate and with pricking sensations.

Phytolacca when the neck is swollen and tender as well as the tonsils – the so-called 'bull neck'.

Sulphur when the tonsils remain large in between attacks, almost touching in the midline; for children who are noticeably 'warm blooded', in contrast to those who need Calc. Carb.

TOOTHACHE

Apis   with swelling of the gums.

Bryonia   when the teeth feel too long.

Calc. Carb.   pain worse for cold air or cold drinks.

Calc. Fluor.   when the dental enamel is deficient.

Chamomilla   worse when in bed.

Coffea   better for cold water.

Kali Carb.   worse when eating.

Mag. Phos.   neuralgic pains like little electric shocks.

Plantago   when the teeth are sensitive to touch and cold air.

Pulsatilla   worse for warm drinks, better in the open air.

Staphisagria   when the teeth are blackened and crumbling.

Obviously, any homoeopathic first aid should be followed by a visit to the dentist.

TRACHEITIS

Apis   with a sensation of swelling in the trachea.

Arsenicum Album   dry, burning and irritating, as if constricted.

Bryonia   worse for talking, smoking and in warm rooms.

Calc. Carb   dry tracheitis, worse in the evening and when speaking.

Cannabis Sativa   worse in the morning, with sticky mucus.

Capsicum   crawling and tickling in the trachea causing sneezing as well as coughing.

Carbo Veg.   worse in the evening.

Causticum   tearing sensations on coughing.

Kali Bich.   irritation in the nose, larynx and trachea, with stringy mucus.

Lachesis   worse after sleep and when touched.

Nux Vomica   tickling, worse when exhaling.

Phosphorus   cough, hawking and rawness, worse in the evening and after cold drinks.

Rumex   soreness worse in cold air.

Silica   mucus coughed up, especially soon after meals.

Stannum   sweetish yellow mucus coughed up.

Sulphur   constant irritation, worse at night.

TRAVEL SICKNESS

This can sometimes be incapacitating, and even dangerous; homoeopathic remedies can control and cure it without causing the drowsiness which is often a side effect of conventional treatment.

Aconite   with restlessness and fear of accident or disaster.

Apomorphine   when vomiting occurs with little or no warning.

Borax   for nausea which is worse during downward movement, as in aircraft, and also in lifts.

Cocculus   almost a specific for travel sickness, especially when there is vertigo and a sense of emptiness in the head.

Petroleum   when nausea is accompanied with eructations of wind from the stomach.

Tabacum   with cold sweat and prostration.

TREMORS

Actea   tremors of the legs, making walking difficult.

Agaricus   rhythmic spasms of groups of muscles, especially of the neck.

Antim. Tart.   tremors of the limbs with coldness of the hands and feet.

Gelsemium   tremors of the whole body, with hot and cold shivers up and down the spine.

Ignatia   tremors combined with gross jerking movements.

Merc. Sol.   tremors of the fingers and of the tongue, with stammering.

Stramonium   tremors persisting after a fright, with writhing movements as well.

ULCERS

This section refers to ulcers of the skin only.

Arsenicum Album   with burning pains, better for warmth.

Belladonna   when the surrounding skin is very red and hot.

Hamamelis   for ulcers associated with varicose veins.

Kali Bich.   when ulcers have a 'punched out' look, with clear-cut edges.

Lachesis   for ulcers with a purple tinge around them.

Merc. Sol.   when there is much oozing of pus and serum.

Mezereum   when scabs form too readily and pus collects under the scabs.

Nitric Acid   for ulcers which bleed easily, and when there are sharp pains like splinters.

Phosphorus   for ulcers which bleed easily.

Silica   when ulcers are slow to develop and slow to heal.

URETHRAL SYNDROME

This section concerns pain on passing urine in the absence of any infection in the bladder, and felt most in the urethra.

Arsenicum Album   burning pain causing agitation – unable to keep still because of the pain.

Camphor   most pain at the beginning of micturition, due to tenesmus at the neck of the bladder.

Clematis   when the urine passes slowly and intermittently, in men more often than in women.

Phosphorus   when urine is passed in small quantities and sometimes with specks of blood.

Sepia   for women more often than for men, and especially for pain due to caruncle.

Silica   when there is urethral stricture.

Terebinth   especially for children when spasms of pain occur just before the urine begins to pass.

URINATION, DISORDERS OF

Apis   burning stinging pain while passing urine, which is scanty and concentrated.

Berberis   when there is mucus in the urine, either as a floating film or as a sediment.

Cantharis   scalding pain and frequency.

Causticum   for frequency in old people, day and night.

Conium   intermittent flow.

Kali Carb.   slow starting, due to prostatic enlargement – helpful while waiting if operation is necessary.

Lilium Tig.   frequent urging and with dragging sensations.

Nux Vomica   for the irritable bladder, in irritable people, resulting in frequency which may be exaggerated.

Petroselinum   sudden urging – any delay causes agony.

URINE, INCONTINENCE OF

This problem occurs mostly in childhood, but also at other ages.

Apis   incontinence with stinging and burning, sometimes as a result of coughing.

Arsenicum Album   during pregnancy.

Belladonna   at night, especially if the urine becomes very concentrated.

Causticum   in old people, who hardly feel the urine passing.

Equisetum   in childhood, at night.

Fluoric Acid   mainly in the daytime.

Merc. Corr.   seems to pass more than is drunk – often associated with tenesmus.

Natrum Mur.   takes more salt than most people.

Phosphoric Acid   as a result of coughing – more in the day than at night.

Pulsatilla   during pregnancy, often while walking.

Sulphur   with burning sensations in the urethra.

URINE, RETENTION OF

Homoeopathic remedies are helpful as first aid, but a surgical opinion will be needed if the trouble persists or recurs.

Apis   when there is oedema of the penis obstructing the urethra.

Arnica   for retention of urine after injury.

Causticum   for retention after surgical operation for any abdominal trouble.

Natrum Mur.   for the patient who cannot pass urine in the presence of anyone.

Nux Vomica   when there is an urge to pass urine every few minutes, but no success.

Opium   retention of urine with no pain and no desire to empty the bladder.

Tarentula   when the patient cannot sit still and relax and allow the urine to flow.

URTICARIA

Acute cases are best treated with **Apis** if the lesions are mainly on the face, or by **Urtica** if the lesions are on the limbs.

Apis burning and stinging, especially with oedema of the eyelids and the lips.

Croton when there is more itching than burning, especially of the genitals, male or female.

Dulcamara for urticaria involving mainly the lower half of the body.

Lycopodium for chronic or persistent urticaria, worse between 4 p.m. and 8 p.m.

Natrum Mur. when the lesions develop after strenuous exercise.

Nux Vomica with mental irritability and intolerance, leading to much scratching.

Rhus Tox. burning and itching, sometimes with vesicles.

Rumex worse when undressing.

Ruta when there is dyspepsia as well as urticaria.

Sulphuric Acid if accompanied by the typical soreness of acid burns.

Urtica for true nettle rash, but also valuable as first aid for urticaria due to other plants.

UTERINE PROLAPSE

This condition usually needs surgical treatment or some form of support. Homoeopathy is often helpful.

Arctium Lappa for prolapse with much bearing-down sensation.

Argentum Nit. when there is ulceration, which needs other treatment as well.

Calc. Carb. when noticably worse after lifting things.

Lilium Tig. 'hurried and worried' – the typical mother and housewife.

Kali Carb. with much backache, especially since the birth of a baby.

Palladium better during social occasions and worse after.

Platinum for prolapse with associated cramps and spasms, especially in haughty superior persons.

Pulsatilla when prolapse is felt more during menstruation.

Sepia the remedy most often indicated for prolapse, with dragging sensations, worse after washing clothes or bathing children, and consequent depression.

VARICOSE VEINS

In addition to support stockings, adequate rest and elevation, and other measures, think of these remedies:

Arnica   when the veins have been bruised or feel bruised.

Calc. Carb.   when the patient is over-weight, chilly, subject to cramps in the calves and feet.

Carbo Veg.   when the peripheral circulation is sluggish, even to the extent of cyanosis.

Fluoric Acid   one of the principal remedies for varicose veins, especially if they are tender and 'knotty'.

Hamamelis   for varicose veins associated with haemorrhoids.

Pulsatilla   particularly useful during pregnancy, when some degree of pelvic pressure impedes the venous circulation.

VERTIGO

This section refers to true vertigo with a rotatory sensation, not to mere faintness.

Belladonna   worse when turning in bed.

Borax   with fear of downward movement.

Bryonia   with vomiting – better keeping still.

Calc. Carb.   worse when looking up.

China Offic.   with tinnitus and debility.

Cocculus   for vertigo associated with travel sickness.

Conium   worse when lying down.

Gelsemium   with trembling.

Kali Carb.   better in the open air.

Natrum Mur.   with headache.

Nux Vomica   with nausea.

Pulsatilla   with catarrh.

VOMITING

This is a symptom of many different causes, and if it persists an accurate diagnosis must be made. As first aid and while waiting for investigations:

Aethusa   when babies or children cannot digest milk without vomiting – different from mere regurgitation.

Antim. Tart.   with much rattling bronchial catarrh which is swallowed and then vomited.

Arsenicum Album   for simultaneous vomiting and diarrhoea.

Cuprum Met.   when vomiting is accompanied by spasms and cramps in the abdominal muscles.

Ipecacuanha   when nausea persists after vomiting, especially during pregnancy.

Iris   for watery vomiting accompanying migraine.

Nux Vomica   if vomiting occurs two or three hours after meals.

Pulsatilla   after rich and fatty foods.

Sulphur   with hot sensations in the chest – retrosternal.

Another helpful approach to the problem of selecting the remedy can be based on the following sections:

Due to **Anger**   Chamomilla, Colocynth, Nux Vomica.

Due to **Cough**   Aluminium, Antim. Tart., Bryonia, Drosera, Hepar Sul., Ipecacuanha, Kali Carb.

With or alternating with **Diarrhoea**   Argentum Nit., Arsenicum Album, Veratrum Album.

After any **Drink**   Antim. Crud., Arsenicum Album, Bryonia, Phosphorus, Tabacum, Veratrum Album.

After only a little **Food**   China Offic., Ipecacuanha, Phosphorus, Sepia, Silica, Sulphur.

With **Headache**   Ipecacuanha, Melilotus, Pulsatilla, Sanguinaria.

During **Pregnancy**   Asarum, Chelidonium, Ignatia, Kreasote, Lactic Acid, Natrum Sul.

Due to **Travelling**   Bryonia, Cocculus Indicus, Petroleum, Tabacum.

WARTS (VERRUCAS)

Calc. Carb.   multiple warts, horny and itchy.

Causticum   multiple warts, especially on the face and on the eyelids.

Dulcamara   large smooth fleshy warts.

Kali Mur.   warts on the hands.

Natrum Carb.   warts which become macerated and ulcerated.

Natrum Mur.   warts on the palms.

Nitric Acid   'cauliflower' warts which itch, prick and bleed easily.

Sepia   large hard pigmented warts.

Sulphur   hard painful warts.

Thuja   the most useful remedy for warts in general, almost a specific.

WHITLOW

Infections around the finger nails can lead to some deformity if they are neglected. In addition to the usual nursing procedures and surgical measures, and antibiotics if necessary, one of the following remedies will be valuable treatment:

Belladonna   when the finger is very hot and throbbing.

Fluoric Acid   if there is a sensation as of a splinter under the nail.

Hepar Sul.   with much throbbing, worse at night and better for holding the hand up.

Lachesis   if there is a blue or purple tinge surrounding the infection.

Silica   when the infection is relatively slow in developing.

WHOOPING COUGH

Antim. Tart. when there is much catarrh, causing 'rattling' sounds in the chest.

Arnica when the child cries out because of the pain of coughing.

Coccus. Cacti when the sputum is stringy, hanging from the mouth in lengths.

Cuprum Met. when there are cramps and even convulsions, as happens sometimes in babies.

Drosera when the cough is worse after midnight.

Hepar Sul. when the paroxysms of coughing are brought on by draughts.

Ipecacuanha when gagging and vomiting follows the coughing.

Kali Carb. when the patient is left exhausted by the cough.

Spongia when the cough sounds rather like a dog barking.

In addition, the nosode, **Pertussin**, is valuable as prophylaxis and also for sequelae, if convalescence is slow.

WOUNDS AND OTHER INJURIES

Arnica for bruises.

Calendula for abrasions and grazes, to encourage the regrowth of the epithelium.

Cantharis for burns and scalds.

Hepar Sul. for wounds and injuries which develop infection.

Hypericum for crush injuries involving damage to nerves, especially of the fingers and toes.

Ledum for puncture wounds – insect stings, needle pricks and stab wounds by wood, metal or other substances.

Rhus Tox. for muscle injuries causing much stiffness.

Staphisagria for pain persisting in surgical wounds.

Symphytum for encouraging union of fractures.

APPENDIX – OUTLINE DESCRIPTIONS OF THE MOST IMPORTANT CONSTITUTIONAL REMEDIES

Dr Marion Gray, BM, BCh, MRCGP, MFHom

This Appendix is provided to enable the reader to identify certain salient characteristics of a patient's total personality, or 'constitution'. This comprises a combination of the physical type, the psychological features, and the reactions to the environment and events.

The personality patterns and the diseases to which they are prone are described under the name of the remedies. It is commonplace in homoeopathy for a patient to be described by the constitutional remedy which most closely suits his or her personality (e.g. a 'Sulphur type', or a 'Sepia type').

Each remedy on the following pages is described in a standard form for ease of reference. First there is a general description of the personality, then a few of the more important modalities (factors which make the condition better or worse). This is followed by typical likes and dislikes of food and drink. Finally, there is a list of the clinical diagnoses indicating the main range of action, provided the complete personality picture conforms.

In general, the constitutional remedies should be used for chronic or recurring diseases. It may happen, for example, that Belladonna is successfully prescribed for a single case of acute otitis media. However, if the child suffers from several episodes of this infection, a constitutional remedy should be sought to prevent further trouble.

It should be stressed that only the most basic information has been provided here to suggest the most likely remedy. It may well be necessary to confirm the choice by reference to a detailed textbook of homoeopathic materia medica.

ARGENTUM NITRICUM
(Nitrate of silver)

This remedy suits anxious thin people who look prematurely aged. Apprehension is a prominent feature.

Warm

But there is an intolerance of heat and a craving for fresh air.

Modalities	**Food**
Better for open air.	Likes sugar.
Worse for mental exertion.	Likes salt.
	Likes cold drinks.
	Likes cheese.

Conditions in which indicated

Gastro-intestinal – flatulent dyspepsia; diarrhoea (like chopped spinach).

Headache – congestive – worse for mental exertion; better for pressure or a tight bandage.

Trembling – sense of imbalance with weakness in the lower limbs.

Apprehensive fears – examination funk; fear of flying; fear of crowded or closed-in places. These may be accompanied by sweating or palpitations, or both.

Splinter-like sensation in the throat.

Eyestrain.

ARSENICUM ALBUM
(Arsenic trioxide)

These patients are usually anxious, pale, thin individuals. They are very sensitive and fastidious. They are also intelligent and quick in mind and body. If ill, their prostration is out of proportion to their condition, and often accompanied by irritability. Their pains are burning in nature.

Chilly   **Right-sided**

Modalities	**Food**
Better for heat.	Wants frequent small drinks.
Worse soon after midnight.	Likes fat.

Conditions in which indicated

Acute colds – fluent watery discharge from the nose causing a sore upper lip.

Diarrhoea and vomiting – especially if occurring at the same time.

Asthma.

Acute heart failure – especially at the early stage.

CALC. CARB.
(Natural calcium carbonate from the middle layer of oyster shells)

These patients are flabby persons who sweat easily on the head and chest. They tend to get depressed easily, and are slow both mentally and physically. They worry a great deal and are forgetful. They even fear that they might lose their reason.

Chilly

Modalities	**Food**
Dislikes open air.	Dislikes milk.
Worse for cold.	Enjoys eggs.

Conditions in which indicated

Enlarged glands.

Faulty bone development – delayed dentition, exostoses and spurs, rickets.

Depression.

Constipation – feels better when constipated. Unlike the similar remedy Graphites, which feels worse when constipated.

Gallstones.

Rheumatism – often follows Rhus Tox. well.

CAUSTICUM
(Potassium hydrate)

The Causticum patient is a broken down, despondent, anxious person who dislikes mental exertion.

Chilly   **Right-sided**

Modalities	**Food**
Better for damp, warm weather.	Worse for sweet foods.
Worse for cold, dry winds.	Worse for coffee.

Conditions in which indicated

Paralysis of single nerves, e.g. Bell's palsy, Horner's syndrome.

Hoarseness – worse in the morning.

Conditions affecting the jaw and mouth. Pain may be referred to the ear.

Rheumatism – contractures of tendons; stiff necks, especially those brought on by draughts.

Urinary difficulties – stress incontinence, frequency.

Warts – on face and finger tips.

GRAPHITES
(Carbon, black lead)

These people are coarse-featured with a tendency to obesity. Their skin is rough, dry and may be cracked. They are indecisive, timid and startle easily. Depression is a common state of mind. Constipation is frequently found. They sometimes complain of an odd sensation as if they felt a cobweb on their face. They are fat, chilly and have a tendency to constipation.

Chilly

Modalities
Better in the dark.

Food
Worse for seafood and fish.
Worse for meat.
Worse for sweet foods.

Conditions in which indicated
Skin – eczema or rashes with sticky secretions like honey, often behind the ear or at the margins of mucous membranes. There may also be crusting.
Digestion – stomach pains relieved by eating. Digestive symptoms and skin complaints may strangely alternate.
Glands – enlarged.
Nose-bleeds – following flushes.

HEPAR SUL.
(Calcium sulphide. Interior of oyster shells burnt with flowers of sulphur)

These are irritable, touchy, over-sensitive people. They sweat easily, but do not like to uncover themselves, preferring to pull a blanket around themselves.

Chilly

Modalities
Better for warm wet weather.
Worse for touch.
Worse for uncovering.
Worse for cold air.

Food
Likes sour food, pickles and condiments.

Conditions in which indicated
Suppuration – profuse secretions smelling like old cheese, e.g. abscesses, infected ulcers, etc.
Tonsillitis – rapid enlargement of glands; sensation of plug or splinter in the throat; pain may be referred to the ear.
Cough and croup.

IGNATIA
(St Ignatius bean)

The emotional aspects of this remedy are of fundamental importance. These patients are nervous and neurotic. Their mental and physical conditions change rapidly and they often present with what seems a contradictory symptom picture.

Chilly

Modalities
Better for heat.
Worse for grief.
Worse for worry.

Food
Desires sour, acid foods.

Conditions in which indicated
Effects of grief.
Hysteria.
Throat – sensation of a lump in the throat. This is better for swallowing, especially solids.
Headaches – worse for coffee; as if a nail had been driven through the side of the head.

KALI BICH.
(Bichromate of potash)

This remedy is well suited to the fat, chubby, sluggish patients who present with ropey, stringy discharges. Pain is characteristically felt in circumscribed small areas. Alternatively, the pains may migrate and alternate with other symptoms (e.g. stomach pain may alternate with catarrh).

Chilly

Modalities
Better for heat.
Worse around 2 a.m.–3 a.m.
Worse for beer.
Worse for undressing.

Food
Craves beer.
Likes starch and potatoes,
  but these upset.

Conditions in which indicated
Chronic catarrh – with tough stringy discharges and crust formation.
Stomach pain – fullness immediately after eating; worse for beer; may be associated with a punched-out ulcer, e.g. a peptic ulcer.
Rheumatism – pains that wander from one place to another.

KALI CARB.
(Potassium carbonate)

This remedy is well-suited to the patient who is full of fears. It also has an element of irritability and great weakness associated with it. The patient may well express a feeling of failure in life, together with distressing forgetfulness. Physically the Kali Carb. type is flabby and sallow, sometimes with flat feet. The impression is one of weakness and depression.

Chilly   **Right-sided**

Modalities
Better for motion.
Worse for touch and easily startled. Worse at 3 a.m. Worse after coition. Worse lying on the left, and on the painful side.

Food
Likes sweet and starchy foods. Likes acid and sour drinks.

Conditions in which indicated
Lungs – asthma. Cough and pneumonia – pain is independent of respiration, often right sided, worse for pressure, better for leaning forward, dry cough with little sputum.
Headache – bitemporal.
Backache – after pregnancy; before menses.
Digestive – flatulence and distension; worse for ice-cold water.

KALI PHOS.
(Potassium phosphate)

This remedy is especially good for the nerves of thin, dark haired, exhausted neurotics. (All Kali salts are fat except Kali Phos.) These patients hate to be alone and yet are very shy and find they are worse for talking to people. They often feel as if they are going to break down.

Chilly

Modalities   **Food**
Better for motion.   Craves ice-cold water.
Better for heat.   Likes sweet foods.
Worse for food.   Likes sour foods.
Worse for worry.
Worse for exertion.
Worse for excitement.

Conditions in which indicated
Headaches – typically in overworking students; the head is tender to the touch.
Insomnia – in adolescents.

LACHESIS
(Venom of the Surukuku snake)

The person requiring Lachesis is usually very loquacious and excitable. There is often a lot of jealousy and suspicion associated with this remedy. An interesting feature is the inability to tolerate tight clothes around the neck. Another marked feature is the blue or purple colour of any skin disorder.

Warm   **Left-sided**

Modalities
Better for the onset of discharges, e.g. nosebleeds, menstruation. Worse after sleep. Worse for pressure (except headaches).

Food
Craves alcohol. Likes oysters. Likes coffee.

Conditions in which indicated
Sore throats – left-sided; purplish tinge to the throat – often looks less bad than the pain would suggest; worse when swallowing, especially hot fluids; empty swallowing may be more painful than swallowing solids; pain may be referred to the ear.
Hot flushes.
Headaches – hammering; from the effects of the sun (follows glonoine well); better for pressure.
Retinal haemorrhages in diabetes.

LUETICUM
(Syphilitic exudate from a chancre)

Suited to chronic conditions which have responded poorly to other well-indicated remedies. Possible family history of syphilis. The patients are often thin and weak, with a poor memory and many fears, especially of becoming insane. They feel compelled to wash their hands frequently.

Modalities
Better inland and in the mountains. Worse at night.

Food
Craves alcohol. (There is a hereditary tendency to alcoholism.)

Conditions in which indicated
Skin – ulcers on the mouth, nose and genitalia; recurrent crops of abscesses; copper-coloured rash.
Rheumatism – often of the shoulder; the pains increase and decrease gradually; the discomfort causes the sufferer to seek frequent changes in position; pains in the long bones.
Neuralgic headaches – may start at 4 p.m. and get worse until midnight.
Obstinate constipation.

Note. This is a nosode, and a deep-acting remedy. It should be used infrequently, ideally once only. A high potency is generally preferred and is administered as the so-called divided dose (half the supply taken, followed by the other half twelve hours later).

LYCOPODIUM
(Club moss)

These people are usually of a reserved and intellectual disposition, but lack physical stamina. They may be tall and thin, and often have a worried expression on their face which results in a furrowed brow. They are sensitive and conscientious people who, although disliking company, dread total solitude. They are subject to anticipatory fears, and get worried about impending responsibilities and public performances, etc.

Chilly
But dislikes 'stuffy' warmth.

Right-sided

Modalities
Worse 4 p.m.–8 p.m.
Worse for tight clothing.
Worse for over-eating.
Hungry, but easily satiated.

Food
Likes sweet foods.
Likes warm drinks.

Conditions in which indicated
Digestive and liver disorders – flatulence; chronic ulcers.
Respiratory tract – neglected or slowly resolving right-sided pneumonia; post-influenzal debility.
Urine – may have a pink sediment.
Sore throat – right sided (may subsequently go to the left); better for warm drinks and worse for cold drinks.

MEDORRHINUM
(Gonorrhoeal pus)

This remedy suits thin individuals with pale waxy skin. They suffer from a poor memory and certain odd feelings of unreality (as if time passed too slowly, or as if life were unreal, 'like a dream'). They are sensitive people and this quality may amount to clairvoyance. They may sleep on their abdomen or, more strangely, favour a position in which the knees are drawn up to the elbows. A nosode: see note on 'Lueticum'.

Modalities
Better at the seashore.
Better for damp.
Worse from daylight to sunset.
Worse for draughts.

Food
Ravenous hunger even after eating. Unquenchable thirst. Likes stimulants, salt, sweet food, sour food.

Conditions in which indicated
Arthritis – especially of the knuckles.
Nasal catarrh – especially if chronic.
Skin – dry scalp; itching dandruff; herpes of the scalp; ringworm; burning sensation of the hands and feet.
Urinary difficulties – frequent urination at night; nocturnal enuresis (bedwetting); discharge.
Neuralgia of the head – worse during the day and on exposure to light.
Gynaecological – obstinate vaginal discharge; profuse painful periods.
Asthma. Arrested development in children.

MERCURIUS
(Black oxide of mercury)

This remedy is characterised by the offensiveness of all discharges, and is useful for people 'filthy in both mind and body'. They are sweaty (the sweat is oily and may stain the bedclothes), weak and tremulous. The tongue is flabby and shows the imprint of the teeth. There may also be spongy, bleeding gums. Much saliva is produced and there is a metallic taste in the mouth.

Modalities
Worse for sweat.
Worse for the warmth of the bed.
Worse at night.

Food
Thirsty for cold drinks.

Conditions in which indicated
Sore throats – with visible exudate on the tonsils. (In the past it was used for diphtheria.)
Glands – enlarged; mumps.
Diarrhoea – green slime; blood; tenesmus during and after evacuation.
Skin – ulcers; itching and stinging.

NATRUM MUR.
(Common salt)

These patients often have sallow, greasy, spotty complexions, with fine, oily hair. They tend to depression and are unstable and touchy. They hate fuss, but dislike to be ignored.

Chilly

Modalities
Worse at 10 a.m.
Worse by the sea.
Worse in the sun.

Food
Thirsty.
Desires salt.

Conditions in which indicated
Depression.
Headache – hammering; migraines.
After shock and grief.
Skin – acne; herpes; urticaria; eczema, especially around the hair margin on the head.
Palpitations.
Irregular menstruation.

NUX VOMICA
(Poison nut which contains strychnine)

This is the remedy for the irritable patient, who is quarrelsome, hates contradiction and is inclined to get angry. He is hypersensitive to noise, light and smell. He is often an epicurean and connoisseur of wine, and typically leads a sedentary life.

Chilly

Modalities
Better for warmth. Better for being alone. Better in the rain.
Worse in the dry, windy weather. Worse two hours after eating. Worse in the open air. Worse for the sun.

Food
Likes piquant food. Likes fat.

Conditions in which indicated
Gastro-intestinal tract – hiatus hernia; indigestion from over-indulgence; diverticulitis; constipation – frequent ineffectual desire to defaecate; rectal problems, e.g. haemorrhoids.
Onset of common cold – esp. if it starts with a scratchy throat.
Headache – on waking, e.g. 'hangover'; worse after sun.
Backache – acute lumbago – has to sit up to turn over in bed.
Hiccough.

PHOSPHORUS

The Phosphorus individual is intelligent, bright and sensitive. Physically, he is often tall and slender. He is imaginative, and this may lead to certain fears, e.g. the dark, of being alone, thunder, etc.

Chilly   **Right upper and left lower complaints**

Modalities
Better for eating – may have night hunger. Better for warmth, except the head and stomach. Better for rubbing.

Food
Desire for salt and spices. Thirsty for cold drinks – these may be vomited when they become warm in the stomach.

Conditions in which indicated
Haemorrhage – bright red blood, e.g. epistaxis.
Respiratory tract – cough (hard dry); asthma; pneumonia – often right lower lobe, worse lying on unaffected side.
Vomiting – can be useful for vomiting of pregnancy.
Headache – migraines, but appetite is not impaired.

PSORINUM
(Scabies vesicle)

This is useful in chronic cases where a selected remedy fails to relieve a patient, even when it seems well indicated. It is suited to people who lack vitality and who appear dirty and smelly (even after washing). They are pale and sickly, and all discharges are offensive. They suffer from anxiety and depression.

Chilly
The head is very sensitive to cold. Some patients may even wear a cap or hat indoors.

Modalities	**Food**
Worse for cold – they dread the least draught.	Hungry in the middle of the night.
Worse in winter.	Always moaning, except when eating!
Worse for changes in weather.	Coffee disagrees.

Conditions in which indicated
Skin – rough, and cracks easily; itching rash – suppurates easily, worse for the heat of the bed; dry scaly scalp with dry hair; acne.
Headache – chronic and periodic in nature; worse at night and made better by eating.
Hayfever – appearing regularly each year.
Cough – every winter.
Asthma – better for lying down with the arms spread wide apart.
Chronic catarrh.

Psorinum is a nosode. See 'Lueticum' for note on dosage and mode of use.

PULSATILLA
(Wind flower)

This remedy is suited to sandy haired individuals, with a tendency to gaining weight easily. They are shy, gentle people (commonly women) prone to tearfulness and changeable moods.

Chilly
Some authorities say warm. Certainly they are averse to heat.

Modalities	**Food**
Better in the fresh air.	Rich foods and fat disagree.
Better for gentle motion.	Thirstless.
Better for sympathy.	
Worse for a stuffy atmosphere.	

Conditions in which indicated
Catarrh – thick bland yellow or green discharge.
Menstrual problems – menses late at puberty; dysmenorrhoea.
Styes.
Varicose veins.
Skin – eczema; urticaria.
Difficulty controlling micturition, e.g. enuresis.
Arthritis.

SEPIA
(Ink of the cuttlefish)

This remedy is well suited to the depressed, indifferent, worn-out person (usually a woman). The Sepia patient is averse to sympathy and company, yet dreads to be alone. Physically, she is often dark haired and has a rather sallow skin.

Chilly

Modalities
Better for food. Better for sleep. Better for exercise, especially dancing. Enjoys a thunderstorm. Worse for tobacco smoke.

Food
Nausea at the thought of food. Dislikes milk, especially if boiled. Loathes fat. Desires vinegar and sour foods.

Conditions in which indicated
Gynaecological – dragging down sensation in the pelvis, better for sitting with crossed legs; menstrual disturbances; menopausal symptoms, e.g. flushes.
Depression – often associated with the menstrual cycle or menopausal problems.
Headache – migraine; headache over the left eye.
Skin – brown patches; ringworm; herpes; urticaria; falling hair, often with an itchy scaly scalp.

SILICEA
(Flint)

This is well suited to the pale-faced, thin, delicate 'china-doll' type person, with small sweaty hands and feet. The Silicea patient appears gentle and even 'spineless' but can be peculiarly obstinate at times. They panic easily at the thought of responsibility, due largely to their feeling of inadequacy and their dread of failure.

Chilly

Modalities	**Food**
Better for warmth.	Poor appetite.
Better for wrapping up (often tight).	Prefers cold food.
Worse for thought of pins and sharp objects.	Dislikes meat.
Worse for draughts.	Thirsty.

Conditions in which indicated
Boils.
Expulsion of foreign bodies, e.g. splinters.
Disorders of the bones, teeth and nails.
Respiratory tract – chest infections that do not clear up; recurrent problems that originate from pleurisy years back.
Headache – occipital – may travel forwards often to settle over the right eye; better for warmth and being tightly wrapped; may follow mental stress.
Constipation – the 'bashful stool' which is difficult to expel.

STAPHISAGRIA
(Stavesacre)

This remedy is suitable for use in patients in whom complaints arise from suppressed anger and indignation. It is also useful for treating the ill effects of sexual excesses.

Modalities
Worse for touch.
Worse for cold.
Worse for coition.

Food
Likes milk.

Conditions in which indicated
Cystitis – especially honeymoon cystitis.
Post-operative pain, and for pain arising from injuries inflicted by knives.
Headache – from vexation and indignation.
Eyes – recurrent styes and meibomian cysts.
Sexual – increased sexual desire often with impotence; very sensitive vulva.
Eczema.

SULPHUR

The Sulphur patient may either be a lank, lean, dyspeptic person with a predisposition to meditation and philosophy, or an active well-fed lover of life. Whatever the type, cleanliness is not a strong point and he will commonly look dishevelled. He is also selfish and has no regard for others.

Warm
Burnings, especially on the soles of the feet.

Modalities
Better for the open air.
Worse for a bath.
Worse for the heat of the bed.
Worse 11 a.m. – sinking feeling.
Worse for standing.

Food
Always hungry.
Likes fat.
Likes sweet foods.
Thirsty.

Conditions in which indicated
Skin – eczema; boils.
Burning pains.
Diarrhoea – that drives the person out of bed in the morning.
Haemorrhoids.
Catarrh.

THUJA
(Arbor vitae)

Suitable for the heavier person with a dark complexion and black hair. A peculiar characteristic is that individuals who need this remedy sweat on uncovered parts, usually when asleep. Mentally, they suffer from odd fixed ideas, such 'as if the limbs were made of glass' or 'as if a strange person was by his side'. It is a deep-acting remedy and has been used to counter the ill effects of smallpox vaccination.

Chilly

Modalities	**Food**
Worse for the heat of the bed.	Great tea drinker.
Worse in the morning.	Dislikes meat.
Worse at night.	Dislikes potatoes.
Worse for the cold damp air.	Worse for fat.
	Worse for onions.

Conditions in which indicated

Skin – large pedunculated warts that bleed easily; polypi; rash on uncovered parts, worse after scratching.

Chronic nasal catarrh – often green.

Eyes – styes and tumour of the eyelids; scleritis.

Asthma.

Abdomen – flatulence and distension (as if something were living inside; constipation – stool recedes after partial expulsion; diarrhoea – gurgling, explosive and worse in the morning.

Urinary difficulties – cystitis – burning during and after passing urine.

TUBERCULINUM BOVINUM
(Pus from a tubercular abscess or from a
tubercular mesenteric gland)

This is indicated when well-selected remedies fail in a patient with a family history of tuberculosis. It suits tall thin, narrow – chested individuals who tire easily. Persons requiring this remedy have a constant desire for change and travel. They may have an irrational fear of dogs.

Chilly
Sensitive to every change in weather, especially cold damp weather.

Modalities
Better in the open air.
Worse in the evening.
Worse for standing.
Worse for changes in the weather.
Worse before a storm.

Food
Large appetite, but remains thin.
Dislikes meat.
Likes cold milk.

Conditions in which indicated
Intermittent fevers – night sweats (that stain the bed linen yellow).
Headache – periodical – worse for overwork; worse for over-eating.
Enlarged tonsils and adenoids with resulting problems.
Recurrent respiratory tract infections – may be brought on by exposure to cold air.
Skin – Eczema with formation of quantities of white scales; ringworm; crops of small boils in the nose.
Bowel – constipation with large stools alternating with diarrhoea; urgent diarrhoea early in the morning.
Menses – periods may be too early, too profuse and painful; there may be, in other cases, amenorrhoea (no periods).

Tuberculinum Bovinum is a nosode. See 'Lueticum' for note on dosage and mode of use.

The Beaconsfield Homoeopathic Library

Classical Homoeopathy, Dr Margery Blackie, 1986, reprinted 1990 with Repertory. The complete teaching legacy of one of the most important homoeopaths of our time.

0906584140

Everyday Homoeopathy, Dr David Gemmell, 1987. A practical handbook for using homoeopathy in the context of one's own personal and family health care, using readily available remedies. 0906584183

Homoeopathic Prescribing, Dr Noel Pratt, revised 1985. A compact reference book covering 161 common complaints and disorders, with guidance on the choice of the appropriate remedy. 0906584035

Homoeopathy as Art and Science, Dr Elizabeth Wright Hubbard, 1990. The selected writings of one of the foremost modern homoeopaths. 0906584264

Homoeopathy in Practice, Dr Douglas Borland, 1982, reprinted 1988 with Symptom Index. Detailed guidance on the observation of symptoms and the choice of remedies.

090658406X

Insights into Homoeopathy, Dr Frank Bodman, 1990. Homoeopathic approaches to common problems in general medicine and psychiatry. 0906584280

Introduction to Homoeopathic Medicine (2nd Edition), Dr Hamish Boyd, 1989. A formal introductory text, written in categories that are familiar to the medical practitioner.

0906584213

Materia Medica of New Homoeopathic Remedies, Dr. O. A. Julian, paperback edition 1984. Full clinical coverage of 106 new homoeopathic remedies, for use in conjunction with the classical materia medicas. 0906584116

Studies of Homoeopathic Remedies, Dr Douglas Gibson, 1987. Detailed clinical studies of 100 major remedies. Well-known for the uniquely wide range of insights brought to bear on each remedy. 0906584175

Tutorials on Homoeopathy, Dr Donald Foubister, 1989. Detailed studies on a wide range of conditions and remedies.

0906584256

Typology in Homoeopathy, Dr Léon Vannier, 1991 (in production). A study of human types, based on the gods of Antiquity, and the remedies which are relevant to them.

0906584302